Dedicated to

All my inquisite students

Acknowledgement

I extend my heartfelt gratitude to Mrs. Pranali Godase for her invaluable assistance in crafting the text with the help of ChatGPT. Equally, my deep appreciation goes to Mrs. Zeenat Shaikh for her dedication in designing the beautiful cover page. Furthermore, I humbly acknowledge the profound contributions of the esteemed authors whose works I have referred to in creating the contents of this book. Their wisdom has been an endless source of inspiration, and I am truly grateful.

The following textbooks have been referenced in the preparation of this work:

1. Gray's 42nd edition of Anatomy the anatomical basis of clinical practice- Editor-in-Chief Susan Standring- International Edition.
2. Anatomy Regional and Applied- R. J. Last - 7th Edition.
3. B. D. Chourasia's handbook of general anatomy – 4th Edition
4. Lesser Known facts of anatomy – Vishram Singh – (Revealing the hidden secrets of human body)

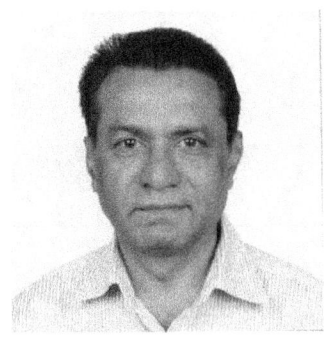

Shoukat N Kazi

Index

Sr.no.	Content	Page no.
1.	Bone	5
2.	Joint	20
3.	Muscle	40
4.	Lymphatic system	67
5.	Cardiovascular system	83
6.	Nervous system	112
7.	Skin and fascia	130
8.	Tissue	178
9.	Endocrine system	199
10.	Genetics and Radiological Anatomy	205
11.	Vertebral column	214
12.	Tendons and ligaments	221

1. Bone

General bone structure and function

Q. 1. Why is bone considered a living tissue despite its rigidity and high calcium content?

Answer: Bone is considered a living tissue because of following reasons:
- It contains blood vessels and
- It has greater reparative power than any other tissue in the body, except blood.

Q. 2. Why is bone described as a strong and rigid connective tissue?

Answer: Bone is described as a strong and rigid connective tissue because of following reasons:
- Bone provides
    - Strength,
    - Support and protection for the body.
- It's not rigidity enables it to create precisely shaped articular surfaces.
- They do not distort under load.
- They ensure rapid limb movements instead of bending.

Q. 3. Why is bone considered highly vascular compared to cartilage?

Answer: Bone is considered highly vascular compared to cartilage because of following reasons:
- It has a high cell density.
- This enables it to adapt to
    - Changing mechanical demands and to
    - Regenerate following injury.

Q. 4. Why do bones display secondary markings?

Answer: Bones display secondary markings mainly in postnatal life because of following reasons:
- Functional adjustments and
- The cumulative effect of
    - Muscle and
    - Ligament pull over time.

- This results in the formation of
    - Elevations,
    - Depressions, and
    - Other surface features.

Q. 5.   Why is vitamin D essential for normal bone development?
Answer: Vitamin D is essential for normal bone development because of following reasons:
- It influences intestinal transport of
    - Calcium and
    - Phosphate, thus affecting circulatory calcium levels.

Q. 6.   Why does bone resorption occur when muscle or gravitational forces are reduced?
Answer: Bone resorption occurs when muscle or gravitational forces are reduced because of following reasons:
- Bones respond to decreased activity by undergoing resorption, as observed in conditions like bed rest or zero gravity.

Q. 7.   Why does the rate of bone remodeling decrease with age?
Answer: The rate of bone remodeling decreases with age because of following reasons:
- Which means that fewer osteons are replaced each year, leading to reduced bone turnover.

Q. 8.   Why do bones provide a rigid framework to the body?
Answer: Bones provide a rigid framework to the body because of following reasons:
- Their mineralized structure
    - Supports and
    - Shapes the body, allowing for
        - Movement and
        - Protection of vital organs.

Q. 9.   Why is the organic material in bones important?
Answer: The organic material, mainly collagen fibers, is important because of following reasons:
- It gives resilience and flexibility to the bones,
- Allowing them to absorb impact without breaking easily.

Q. 10.   Why do bones appear radiopaque in x-ray films?

Answer: Bones appear radiopaque (white or light) on X-ray films because they are dense and absorb more X-rays compared to surrounding tissues.

1. **Bone Density:** Bones are made of minerals like calcium, which are dense and have a higher atomic number. This density means that bones block or absorb more of the X-rays as they pass through the body.

2. **X-ray Interaction:** When X-rays pass through the body, they are absorbed to varying degrees by different tissues. Dense tissues like bones absorb more X-rays, while softer tissues like muscles and fat absorb fewer.
3. **X-ray Film:** On the X-ray film or image, areas where X-rays are absorbed less (like soft tissues) appear darker, while areas where more X-rays are absorbed (like bones) appear lighter or white. This contrast creates the clear images of bones seen on X-rays.

In summary, bones appear radiopaque on X-ray films because their density causes them to absorb more X-rays, preventing those X-rays from reaching the film, which results in a lighter or white appearance.

Q. 11. Why is the ability of bones to regenerate significant?

Answer: The ability of bones to regenerate is significant because of following reasons:
- It allows bones to repair themselves after injury.
- It maintains the structural integrity and function of the skeletal system.

Q. 12. Why do bones have greater regenerative power than most other tissues?

Answer: Bones have greater regenerative power than most other tissues because of following reasons:
- Due to their rich blood supply and
- The presence of bone-forming cells (osteoblasts) that facilitate the repair and regeneration process.

Q. 13. Why is it incorrect to think of bones as inert materials?

Answer: It is incorrect to think of bones as inert materials because of following reasons:
- They are living structures with active cellular processes, including
    - Growth,
    - Remodelling, and
    - Repair, supported by blood vessels, lymph vessels, and nerves.

Q. 14. Why are bones subject to diseases like other tissues?

Answer: Bones are subject to diseases like other tissues because of following reasons:
- They are living structures that can be affected by
    - Infections,
    - Metabolic disorders, and
    - Genetic conditions, impacting their function and integrity.

Q. 15. **Why do bones protect certain viscera like the brain, spinal cord, heart, and lungs?**
Answer: Bones protect certain viscera because these organs are because of following reasons:
Vital and delicate, requiring the rigid protection provided by the skeletal structure to prevent injury.

Q. 16. **Why are bones a storehouse of calcium and phosphorus?**
Answer: Bones are a storehouse of calcium and phosphorus because of following reasons:
- These minerals are essential for various bodily functions, including bone strength and density, and are stored in bones to maintain adequate levels in the body.

Q. 17. **Why do bones indicate a complex interplay of various functions?**
Answer: Bones indicate a complex interplay of various functions because of following reasons:
- They not only provide structural support and movement but also
- Play critical roles in protection,
- Blood cell production,
- Mineral storage, and
- Influencing voice quality.

Q. 18. **Why are bones essential for movement?**
Answer: Bones are essential for movement because of following reasons:
- They act as levers that muscles pull on to create motion, allowing for various physical activities and mobility.

Q. 19. **Why bone is considered a specialized connective tissue?**
Answer: Bone is considered a specialized connective tissue because of following reasons:
- It consists of cells, ground substance, and fibers that
- Matrix,
- Providing structural support and
- Various other functions.

Q. 20. **Why do bones have a basic structure of an outer compact bone and inner spongy bone?**

Answer: Bones have a basic structure of an outer compact bone and inner spongy bone because
- This arrangement provides a balance of following reasons:
    o Strength and
    o Lightness, allowing bones to withstand various stresses while being efficient in weight.

Q. 21. **Why does the growth in length of long bones occur through endochondral ossification?**

Answer: The growth in length of long bones occurs through endochondral ossification because of following reason:
- The process allows continuous production of new cartilage at the epiphyseal plate. It is gradually replaced by bone, enabling longitudinal growth.

Q. 22. **Why does bone include calcium salts?**

Ans: Bone includes calcium salts because of following reason:
- They make it hard and rigid, capable of resisting compressive forces.

Q. 23. **Why is bone compared to iron and steel in terms of strength?**

Ans: Bone is compared to iron and steel in terms of strength because of following reason:
- Its hardness and the organic collagen fibers make it tough and resilient.
- Bone is incredibly strong and can withstand significant forces. Despite being lightweight, bone has a high tensile and compressive strength, similar to that of iron and steel, making it capable of supporting and protecting the body effectively.

Q. 24. **Why are bones of elderly individuals more prone to fractures?**

Ans: Bones of elderly individuals are more prone to fractures because of following reason:
- They contain less collagen and are less dense due to osteoporosis.
- This combination of factors makes the bones brittle and susceptible to breaking under normal stress.

Q. 25. **Why do females stop growing earlier than males?**

Ans: Females stop growing earlier than males because of following reasons:
- Oestrogen hastens the closure of epiphyseal plates, which are responsible for bone growth in length. This hormonal influence leads to earlier cessation of bone lengthening and hence shorter stature in females compared to males.

Compact bone

Q. 26. Why is compact bone immensely strong?
Answer: Compact bone is immensely strong because of following reasons:
- It has collagen fibers contribute rugged elasticity to its stony-hard brittleness.
- Collagen fibres are capable of withstanding crushing pressure.

Q. 27. Why are Haversian systems present in compact bone?
Answer: Haversian systems are present in compact bone to because of following reasons:
- Provide a network of blood vessels and
- Facilitate nutrient exchange within the bone.

Q. 28. Why is compact bone important in determining bone strength?
Answer: Compact bone is important in determining strength of the bone because of following reasons:
- It is usually limited to the outer shell or cortex of mature bones.
- It provides rigid articular surfaces.
- It contributes to overall bone strength.

Q. 29. Why do cortical capillaries follow the pattern of Haversian canals?
Answer: Cortical capillaries follow the pattern of Haversian canals to supply because of following reasons:
- Fenestrated capillaries in Haversian systems and
- Maintain the blood flow within the cortical bone structure.

Q. 30. Why do Haversian canals run parallel to the long axis of the bone?
Answer: Haversian canals run parallel to the long axis of the bone because of following reasons:
- this orientation allows for efficient delivery of nutrients and
- Removal of waste products through the bone's vascular system.

Long bones

Q. 31. Why does the shaft of a long bone provide maximum strength with minimal material and weight?
Answer: The shaft of a long bone provides maximum strength with minimal material and weight because of following reasons:
- It is composed of a thick shell of compact bone surrounding a medullary cavity, optimizing structural efficiency.

Q. 32. **Why is the medullary cavity of a long bone filled with yellow bone marrow in adults?**
Answer: The medullary cavity of a long bone is filled with yellow bone marrow in adults because of following reasons:
- The red bone marrow, which is present at birth, is gradually replaced by yellow marrow as the body ages.

Q. 33. **Why are the ends of long bones covered by articular hyaline cartilage?**
Answer: The ends of long bones are covered by articular hyaline cartilage because of following reasons:
- this cartilage provides a smooth, lubricated surface for joint movement and
- Reduces friction.

Q. 34. **Why can yellow bone marrow convert back into red bone marrow under certain conditions?**
Answer: Yellow bone marrow can convert back into red bone marrow under certain conditions, such as severe bleeding or hypoxia, because of following reasons:
- The body may need to increase blood cell production in response to these stressors.

Q. 35. **Why are epiphyseal plates important for the growth in length of long bones?**
Answer: Epiphyseal plates are important for the growth in length of long bones because of following reasons:
- They are sites of active cell proliferation and cartilage formation.
- They are essential for longitudinal bone growth during development.

Q. 36. **Why does the diaphysis develop from a primary ossification center?**
Answer: The diaphysis develops from a primary ossification center because of following reasons:
- The primary center initiates the process of bone formation.
- It allows the long bone to grow in
    - length and
    - Strength from an early stage of development.

Q. 37. **Why is the metaphysis the most vascular zone of the long bone?**
Answer: The metaphysis is the most vascular zone of the long bone because of the following reasons:
- The nutrient artery divides into numerous smaller vessels in the medullary cavity.

- They form hair-pin loops.
- They anastomose with
    - epiphyseal,
    - metaphyseal, and
    - Periosteal arteries.

Q. 38. **Why does the nutrient artery of the tibia stand out among nutrient arteries?**
Answer: The nutrient artery of the tibia stands out among nutrient arteries because of the following reason:
- It is the largest nutrient artery in the body.
- It supplies significant blood to the tibia.

Q. 39. **Why do periosteal arteries particularly numerous beneath muscular and ligamentous attachments?**
Answer: Periosteal arteries are particularly numerous beneath muscular and ligamentous attachments because of the following reason:
- These areas require a robust blood supply.
- This is to support the high metabolic demands of
    - muscle and
    - Ligament interactions with the bone.

Q. 40. **Why do epiphyseal arteries often pierce the epiphyseal cartilage?**
Answer: Epiphyseal arteries often pierce the epiphyseal cartilage because of the following reasons:
- The blood is directly supplied to the
    - developing and
    - Growing epiphyseal region.
- It is extremely important for proper
    - bone development and
    - Joint function.

Q. 41. **Why is the nutrient artery important for the blood supply of a rib?**
Answer: The nutrient artery is important for the blood supply of a rib because of the following reason:
- it provides the primary blood supply by entering the rib just behind the tubercle,
- It ensures that the bone receives adequate nutrients and oxygen.

Flat bones

Q. 42.   **Why do flat bones form the boundaries of certain body cavities?**
Answer: Flat bones form the boundaries of certain body cavities because of following reasons:
- Their broad, flat surfaces provide protection and support for vital organs.

Irregular bones

Q. 43.   **Why are irregular bones highly irregular in shape?**
Answer: Irregular bones are highly irregular in shape because of following reasons:
- Their complex forms are adapted to their
    - Specific functions and
    - Locations, such as providing
        - Support and
        - Protection for different parts of the body.

Sesamoid bones

Q. 44.   **Why do sesamoid bones develop in muscle tendons?**
Answer: Sesamoid bones develop in muscle tendons because of following reasons:
- They reduce friction, alter the direction of muscle pull, and
- Act as pulleys for muscle contraction.

Pneumatic bones

Q. 45.   **Why do certain irregular bones contain large air spaces lined by epithelium?**
Ans: Certain irregular bones contain large air spaces lined by epithelium because of following reasons:
- To reduce weight,
- Aid in voice resonance, and
- Act as air conditioning chambers for inspired air.

Short bones

Q. 46.　Why are short bones supplied by numerous fine vessels from the periosteum?
Answer: Short bones are supplied by numerous fine vessels from the periosteum because of following reasons:
  To supply both
- Compact and
- Cancellous bone, as well as
- Medullary cavities, ensuring sufficient blood flow for their metabolic needs.

Q. 47.　Why are short bones usually cuboidal in shape?
Answer: Short bones are usually cuboidal in shape because of following reasons:
- This shape allows them to provide
  - Stability and
  - Support with little to no movement.

Accessory bones

Q. 48.　Why are accessory bones sometimes mistaken for fractured bones?
Answer: Accessory bones are sometimes mistaken for fractured bones because of following reasons:
- They are extra bones that are not typically present,
- And their appearance can resemble bone fragments seen in fractures.

Q. 49.　Why are accessory (supernumerary) bones not always present?
Ans: Accessory (supernumerary) bones are not always present because of following reasons:
- They may occur as ununited epiphyses from extra centers of ossification, and they can be mistaken for fractures in medico legal practice.

Bone marrow

Q. 50.　Why does marrow in long bones change from red to yellow as age advances?
Answer: Marrow in long bones changes from red to yellow as age advances because of following reasons:
- Red marrow atrophies and is replaced by yellow, fatty marrow, with no hematopoietic function.

Q. 51. **Why is bone marrow important for the production of blood cells?**
Answer: Bone marrow is important for the production of blood cells because of following reasons:
- It is the primary site for the generation of white blood cells, red blood cells, and platelets, which are crucial for immune function, oxygen transport, and blood clotting.

Periosteum and blood supply

Q. 52. **Why does the periosteum play a crucial role in bone nutrition and repair?**
Answer: The periosteum plays a crucial role in bone nutrition and repair because of following reasons:
- It contains blood vessels and osteogenic cells that can differentiate into osteoblasts for bone formation and repair.

Q. 53. **Why do one or two main diaphyseal nutrient arteries enter the shaft obliquely through nutrient foramina?**
Answer: One or two main diaphyseal nutrient arteries enter the shaft obliquely through nutrient foramina because of following reasons:
- To supply blood to the bone tissue, marrow, perichondrium, and epiphysial cartilages, and they are almost constant and characteristically directed away from the dominant growing epiphysis.

Q. 54. **Why do medullary arteries in the shaft give off centripetal branches?**
Answer: Medullary arteries in the shaft give off centripetal branches to feed a hexagonal mesh of medullary sinusoids that drain into a wide, thin-walled central venous sinus, ensuring adequate blood supply to the bone tissue.

Q. 55. **Why are periosteal arteries crucial for the overall blood supply to bones?**
Answer: Periosteal arteries are crucial for the overall blood supply to bones because of following reasons:
- They supply the outer one-third of the cortex, supporting the bone's outer structure and facilitating the attachment of muscles and ligaments.

Q. 56. **Why are endosteal vessels vulnerable during surgical operations such as intramedullary nailing?**
Answer: Endosteal vessels are vulnerable during surgical operations such as intramedullary nailing because of following reasons:
- These operations involve passing metal implants into the medullary canal, which can potentially damage these vessels.

Q. 57. **Why is the arterial supply richer in epiphysial and metaphysial regions compared to diaphyseal regions?**
Answer: The arterial supply is richer in epiphysial and metaphysial regions compared to diaphyseal regions because of following reasons:
- The epiphysial and metaphysial arterial supply is supported by numerous branches from neighboring systemic vessels and peri-articular vascular arcades, providing a more extensive blood supply.

Bone cells:

Q. 58. **Why are osteoblasts important in bone formation?**
Answer: Osteoblasts are important in bone formation because of following reasons:
- They secrete osteoid, which later mineralizes to become bone, and release essential factors like osteocalcin and alkaline phosphatase that facilitate mineralization.

Q. 59. **Why do osteoblasts secrete osteocalcin and alkaline phosphatase?**
Answer: Osteoblasts secrete osteocalcin and alkaline phosphatase because of following reasons:
- To release calcium and phosphate radicals necessary for the mineralization of the bone matrix.

Q. 60. **Why are osteocytes derived from osteoblasts?**
Answer: Osteocytes are derived from osteoblasts because of following reasons:
- Once osteoblasts become surrounded by the matrix they secrete, they transform into osteocytes, residing in lacunae within the bone matrix.

Q. 61. **Why do osteocytes not undergo mitosis?**
Answer: Osteocytes do not undergo mitosis because their primary function is to maintain the bone matrix rather than proliferate, unlike osteoblasts which are involved in the active formation of bone.

Q. 62. **Why are canaliculi important for osteocytes?**
Answer: Canaliculi are important for osteocytes because they allow the diffusion of nutrients and waste products, keeping the osteocytes alive within the calcified matrix and maintaining bone health.

Q. 63.   **Why are osteoclasts crucial for bone remodeling?**
Answer: Osteoclasts are crucial for bone remodeling because they resorb bone tissue, allowing for the removal of old or damaged bone and facilitating the formation of new bone.

Q. 64.   **Why do osteoclasts reside in How ship's lacunae?**
Answer: Osteoclasts reside in how ship's lacunae because these shallow depressions in the bone surface are sites where they actively break down bone tissue during resorption.

Q. 65.   **Why are osteoblasts responsible for bone matrix synthesis and mineralization?**
Answer: Osteoblasts are responsible for bone matrix synthesis and mineralization because they synthesize and secrete collagen and other organic components of the bone matrix, which then mineralize to form bone tissue.

Ossification and bone development

Q. 66.   **Why are certain bones, like those of the cranial vault, formed through intramembranous ossification?**
Answer: Bones of the cranial vault are formed through intramembranous ossification because they are laid down in a fibro-cellular membrane of mesenchyme, where osteoblasts differentiate directly from mesenchymal templates.

Q. 67.   **Why do osteoblasts become trapped in the organic material they secrete during ossification?**
Answer: Osteoblasts become trapped in the organic material they secrete during ossification because as they secrete organic material, they become surrounded by it, forming what are called osteocytes, which are embedded within the bone matrix.

Q. 68.   **Why is the bone formed in Step 3 of ossification referred to as "woven bone"?**
Answer: The bone formed in Step 3 of ossification is referred to as "woven bone" because the collagen fibers in this type of bone are arranged randomly, resembling the crisscross pattern of woven fabric.

Q. 69.   **Why is woven bone seen only during fetal development and in the repair of fractures?**
Answer: Woven bone is seen only during fetal development and in the repair of fractures because it is an immature form of bone that is quickly laid down to provide structural support during early development or as a temporary measure during healing.

Q. 70.   **Why are all adult bones, whether cancellous or compact, classified as lamellar bones?**

Answer: All adult bones, whether cancellous (spongy) or compact (dense), are classified as lamellar bones because they are characterized by their mature structure, where the collagen fibers are organized into layers called lamellae.

Q. 71.   **Why intramembranous ossification is clinically less important compared to endochondral ossification?**

Answer: Intramembranous ossification is clinically less important compared to endochondral ossification because it primarily forms flat bones and the clavicle, whereas endochondral ossification is responsible for the formation of all long bones and many other bones critical for skeletal support and movement.

Q. 72.   **Why does the appearance of secondary centers of ossification occur after birth?**

Answer: The appearance of secondary centres of ossification occurs after birth because they are responsible for the formation of the epiphyses of long bones, which continue to grow and develop after birth until the epiphyses fuse with the diaphysis.

Q. 73.   **Why does the fusion of epiphyses with the diaphysis start at puberty?**

Answer: The fusion of epiphyses with the diaphysis starts at puberty because hormonal changes at this time signal the end of longitudinal bone growth, leading to the closure of the epiphyseal plates and the cessation of bone lengthening.

Miscellaneous questions

Q. 74.   **Why are nerves most numerous in periosteum, articular extremities, vertebrae, and larger flat bones?**

Answer: Nerves are most numerous in periosteum, articular extremities, vertebrae, and larger flat bones to provide sensory innervation and feedback, especially in areas where mechanical stress and strain are common.

Q. 75.   **Why do some bones around the nose contain large cavities filled with air?**

Answer: Some bones around the nose contain large cavities filled with air, known as paranasal sinuses, because they help to reduce the weight of the skull and affect the resonance and timbre of the voice.

Q. 76. **Why does postnatal growth and maintenance of bone modelling occur in all growing bones?**
Answer: Postnatal growth and maintenance of bone modelling occur in all growing bones to accommodate changes in general shape.

Q. 77. **Why does the rate of bone formation increase with radial distance from the center of ossification?**
Answer: The rate of bone formation increases with radial distance from the center of ossification to accommodate growth and expansion, particularly in areas like the future parietal eminence.

Q. 78. **Why does osteomyelitis in the metaphysis become rare in adults?**
Answer: Osteomyelitis in the metaphysis becomes rare in adults because, after epiphyseal fusion, the metaphyseal arteries establish communications with epiphyseal arteries, reducing the presence of end arteries and thus the likelihood of infections.

Q. 79. **Why do tendons attach at roughened bone surfaces?**
Answer: Tendons attach at roughened bone surfaces because the roughness provides a better grip and stability for tendon attachment, ensuring efficient transmission of forces between muscles and bones.

Q. 80. **Why are surface markings on bones important?**
Answer: Surface markings on bones are important because they delineate the shape of attached connective tissue structures such as tendons, ligaments, and muscles, providing accurate indications of bone-muscle and bone-ligament junctions.

Q. 81. **Why do heterotopic bones sometimes develop in soft tissues?**
Answer: Heterotopic bones sometimes develop in soft tissues, such as in the adductor muscles of horse riders (rider's bones), due to chronic stress or trauma.

2. Joints

Fibrous Joints

Q. 1. Why are fibrous joints classified into 3 subtypes?

Answer: Fibrous joints are classified into 3 subtypes that are as follow:

- Sutures,
- Gomphoses,
- Syndesmoses
  Bones in fibrous joints are joined by fibrous connective tissue. They allow little movement, and these subtypes represent different types of fibrous connections between bones.

Q. 2. Why do sutures synostose and become obliterated after completion of growth?

Answer: Sutures synostose and become obliterated after completion of growth because of following reasons.

- The region between the capsular coverings contains loose fibrous connective tissue.
- It decreases with age, causing the osteogenic surfaces to become apposed.

Q. 3. Why a gomphosis is not strictly considered an articulation between 2 skeletal structures?

Answer: A gomphosis is not strictly considered an articulation between 2 skeletal structures because of following reasons.

- It is a peg-and-socket junction between a tooth and its socket.
- Here the 2 components are maintained in intimate contact by the collagen of the periodontium called periodontal membrane. It connects the dental cement to the alveolar bone.

Q. 4. Why can a syndesmosis be represented by various fibrous connections between bones?

Answer: A syndesmosis can be represented by various fibrous connections between bones because of following reasons.

- It may be represented by
  - An interosseous ligament, a slender fibrous cord, or
  - A denser fibrous membrane, depending on the specific joint.

Q. 5. Why are fibrous joints immobile and strong?

Answer: Fibrous joints are immobile and strong because of following reason:

- The surfaces are joined simply by fibrous tissue.
- The degree of movement depends on the area of the joint surface and the length of the uniting fibers.

Q. 6.   Why are sutures classified as immovable joints?
Answer: Sutures are classified as immovable joints because of following reasons:
- They are peculiar to the skull and the bones are joined tightly by fibrous tissue.
- These joints do not permit movement to protect the brain and support the skull structure.

Q. 7.   Why are sutures grouped into different subtypes?
Answer: Sutures are grouped into different subtypes because of following reasons:
- Based on the shape of their bony margins.
- This classification helps in understanding their specific anatomical features and functions.

Q. 8.   Why the syndesmosis is joint considered a fibrous joint?
Answer: The syndesmosis joint is considered a fibrous joint because of following reasons:
- The bones are connected by the interosseous ligament.
- It is a type of fibrous connective tissue.

Q. 9.   Why the gomphosis is joint referred to as a peg and socket joint?
Answer: The gomphosis joint is referred to as a peg and socket joint because of following reasons:
- It involves the root of a tooth fitting into its bony socket
- Resembling a peg inserted into a socket.

Q. 10.   Why are cranial sutures in adults classified as immovable joints (synarthroses)?
Answer: Cranial sutures in adults are classified as immovable joints (synarthroses) because of following reasons:
- They provide stability and protect the brain by forming a rigid structure.

Q. 11.   Why do secondary cartilaginous joints and syndesmoses fall under slightly movable joints (amphiarthroses)?
Answer: Secondary cartilaginous joints and syndesmoses fall under slightly movable joints (amphiarthroses) because of following reasons:
- They allow for some degree of flexibility and movement
- Which is essential for certain functions and movements in the body.

Q. 12.   Why are sutures classified as fibrous joints?
Answer: Sutures are classified as fibrous joints because of following reasons:
- The bones are united by a thin layer of connective tissue, providing a rigid and immovable connection.

Q. 13.   **Why does Gardner's observation highlight the innervation pattern of joint capsules by nerves that also supply antagonistic muscles?**

Answer: Gardner's observation highlight the innervation pattern of joint capsules by nerves that also supply antagonistic muscles because of following reasons:
- This arrangement establishes local reflex arcs, ensuring joint stability through coordinated muscle actions.

Cartilaginous Joints

Q. 14.   **Why are cartilaginous joints classified as primary or secondary?**

Answer: Cartilaginous joints are classified as primary or secondary because of following reasons.
- It depends upon the type of cartilage separating 2 bones. Primary cartilaginous joints the bones are separated by hyaline cartilage.
- Secondary joints is characterized by a fibrocartilage which separates 2 which separates 2 articular cartilage.

Q. 15.   **Why do synchondroses tend to synostose when growth is complete?**

Answer: Synchondroses tend to synostose when growth is complete because of following reasons.
- Hyaline cartilage retains the capability to ossify with age, leading to the fusion of advancing centers of ossification separated by the cartilage.

Q. 16.   **Why all epiphyses are considered primary cartilaginous joints?**
Answer: All epiphyses are considered primary cartilaginous joints because of following reason:
- They involve the junction of bone and hyaline cartilage, making them immobile and strong.

Q. 17.   **Why are secondary cartilaginous joints also known as symphyses?**
Answer: Secondary cartilaginous joints are also known as symphyses because of following reason:
- They involve a union between bones with articular surfaces covered by a thin layer of hyaline cartilage,
- Which is united by fibro-cartilage.

Q. 18. **Why do some secondary cartilaginous joints allow limited movement?**
Answer: Some secondary cartilaginous joints allow limited movement because of following reason:
- They are composed of fibrocartilage, which is flexible and can compress slightly.
- This structure provides both stability and a small range of movement.
- These joints are suited for areas that endure pressure but need some flexibility. For example, the intervertebral discs in the spine have this feature.

Q. 19. **Why primary cartilaginous joints are considered immovable and strong?**
Answer: Primary cartilaginous joints are considered immovable and strong because of following reasons:
- The bones are united by a plate of hyaline cartilage
- Which provides stability and strength.

Q. 20. **Why are primary cartilaginous joints temporary in nature?**
Answer: Primary cartilaginous joints are temporary because of following reasons:
- After a certain age, the cartilaginous plate is replaced by bone through a process called synostosis.

Q. 21. **Why do secondary cartilaginous joints permit limited movements?**
Answer: Secondary cartilaginous joints permit limited movements because of following reasons:
- They have a disc of fibrocartilage between the articular surfaces
- The disc is compressible and allows slight movement.

Q. 22. **Why the symphysis menti is considered a misnomer?**
Answer: The symphysis menti is considered a misnomer because of following reasons:
- Unlike other secondary cartilaginous joints, it is a synostosis, meaning the cartilage has been replaced by bone.

Q. 23. **Why do secondary cartilaginous joints typically occur in the median plane of the body?**
Answer: Secondary cartilaginous joints typically occur in the median plane of the body because of following reasons:
- This central positioning allows for balanced and limited movements essential for stability and function.

Q. 24. **Why the thickness of fibrocartilage in secondary cartilaginous joints is directly related to the range of movement?**
Answer: The thickness of fibrocartilage in secondary cartilaginous joints is directly related to the range of movement because of following reasons:
- Thicker fibrocartilage can compress more, allowing for greater movement.

Q. 25.   **Why might secondary cartilaginous joints represent an intermediate stage in the evolution of synovial joints?**

Answer: Secondary cartilaginous joints might represent an intermediate stage in the evolution of synovial joints because of following reasons:
- They combine features of both rigid and movable joints, indicating a transitional form.

Q. 26.   **Why synchondroses are considered primary cartilaginous joints?**

Answer: Synchondroses are considered primary cartilaginous joints because of following reasons:
- The bones are joined by a plate of hyaline cartilage, which is eventually replaced by bone as the individual grows.

Q. 27.   **Why are symphyses classified as secondary cartilaginous joints?**

Answer: Symphyses are classified as secondary cartilaginous joints because of following reasons:
- The bones are connected by fibrocartilage pads, allowing for slight movement while maintaining stability.

Synovial Joints

Q. 28.   **Why are synovial joints classified as freely moving joints?**

Answer: Synovial joints are classified as freely moving joints because of following reasons.
- The articulating bony surfaces are covered smooth (hyaline) articular cartilage.
- They are separated by a film of viscous synovial fluid that serves as a lubricant. It allows a wide range of movement between bones.

Q. 29.   **Why is joint stability provided by a fibrous capsule in synovial joints?**

Answer: Joint stability is provided by a fibrous capsule in synovial joints because of following reasons.
- The capsule completely encloses each joint except where it is interrupted by synovial protrusions.
- It is composed of interlacing bundles of parallel fibers of collagen type
- They are attached continuously round the ends of the articulating bones.

Q. 30.   **Why does synovial membrane secrete and absorb synovial fluid?**

Answer: Synovial membrane secretes and absorbs synovial fluid because of following reasons.
- It provides lubrication to the articulating surfaces.
- It provides the nutrition to the cells in the articular cartilages.

Q. 31. **Why should the term "meniscus" be reserved for incomplete discs, like those in the knee joint?**

Answer: The term "meniscus" should be reserved for incomplete discs because of following reasons.

- They occur in areas where congruity between opposing articular surfaces is low.

Q. 32. **Why are complete discs, such as those in the sternoclavicular and inferior radio-ulnar joints, structurally divided into 2 synovial cavities?**

Answer: Complete discs are structurally divided into 2 synovial cavities because of following reasons:

- They extend across a synovial joint.

Q. 33. **Why do joints that contain an intra-articular disc or meniscus classified as complex joints?**

Answer: Joints that contain an intra-articular disc or meniscus are classified as complex joints because of following reason:

- The articular disc or meniscus in synovial joint influence biomechanics and function. Therefore they are called as complex joint.

Q. 34. **Why do synovial joints have different degrees of freedom?**

Answer: Synovial joints have different degrees of freedom because of following reason:

- It depends on the
    - Complexity of their articulating surfaces and
    - The number of principal axes of movement.

Q. 35. **Why do some synovial joints have one degree of freedom while others have up to three degrees of freedom?**

Answer: Some synovial joints have one degree of freedom while others have up to three degrees of freedom because of following reason:

- Their movement is practically limited to rotation about one axis,
- They can rotate around multiple axes.

Q. 36. **Why do ligaments composed of elastic tissue contribute differently to joint stability compared to ligaments composed of collagen fibers?**

Answer: Ligaments composed of elastic tissue contribute differently to joint stability because of following reasons:

- They can shorten after elongation,
- Whereas ligaments composed of collagen fibers tend to remain elongated once stretched.

Q. 37. Why are diarthroses classified as freely movable joints, like synovial joints?
Answer: Diarthroses are classified as freely movable joints, like synovial joints because of following reasons:
- They have a synovial cavity filled with synovial fluid which allows for a wide range of movements.
- Examples include the knee and shoulder joints.

Q. 38. Why is the vertebral type of joint classified as slightly movable?
Answer: The vertebral type of joint is classified as slightly movable because of following reasons:
- There is limited movement due to the presence of intervertebral discs.
- There is some flexibility allowed by the ligaments between the vertebrae.

Q. 39. Why do synovial joints facilitate a wide range of movements?
Answer: Synovial joints facilitate a wide range of movements because of following reasons:
- They have a joint cavity filled with synovial fluid
- Which reduces friction and allows for smooth articulation between bones.

Q. 40. Why are synovial joints classified as diarthrodial joints?
Answer: Synovial joints are classified as diarthrodial joints because of following reasons:
- They are the most evolved and allow for the greatest range of movement.

Q. 41. Why do synovial joints have a joint cavity filled with synovial fluid?
Answer: Synovial joints have a joint cavity filled with synovial fluid because of following reasons:
- To lubricate the articular surfaces and provide nutrition to the articular cartilages.

Q. 42. Why are articular surfaces in synovial joints covered by hyaline cartilage?
Answer: Articular surfaces in synovial joints are covered by hyaline cartilage because of following reasons:
- To ensure smooth and frictionless movement of the joint.

Q. 43. Why is the synovial membrane important in synovial joints?
Answer: The synovial membrane is important in synovial joints because of following reasons:
- It secretes synovial fluid, which lubricates and nourishes the joint.

Q. 44. **Why do articular discs or menisci prevent wear and tear of articular cartilages?**
Answer: Articular discs or menisci prevent wear and tear of articular cartilages because of following reasons:
- By providing a cushioning effect between the articular surfaces.

Q. 45. **Why do bursae reduce the friction of structures moving over each other near synovial joints?**
Answer: Bursae reduce the friction of structures moving over each other near synovial joints because of following reasons:
- Providing a cushion filled with synovial fluid, facilitating smooth movement.

Q. 46. **Why do plane joints permit gliding movements in various directions?**
Answer: Plane joints permit gliding movements in various directions because of following reasons:
- Their articular surfaces are nearly flat, allowing side-to-side and back-and-forth movements with slight rotation.

Q. 47. **Why are hinge joints limited to movements in one plane around a transverse axis?**
Answer: Hinge joints are limited to movements in one plane around a transverse axis because of following reasons:
- Their pulley-shaped articular surfaces and strong collateral ligaments restrict movements to flexion and extension.

Q. 48. **Why do pivot joints allow limited rotation around a central axis?**
Answer: Pivot joints allow limited rotation around a central axis because their structure includes a cylindrical bone that rotates within a ring-like structure. This design restricts movement to rotational only, providing stability and control around the axis.

Q. 49. **Why do condylar joints permit movements in two directions?**
Answer: Condylar joints permit movements in two directions because
- Their structure features an oval-shaped condyle fitting into an elliptical socket. This configuration allows flexion and extension as well as abduction and adduction.

Q. 50. **Why do ellipsoidal joints allow flexion, extension, abduction, and adduction?**
Answer: Ellipsoidal joints allow flexion, extension, abduction, and adduction because of following reasons:
- Their elliptical convex and concave articular surfaces permit movements around two axes, resulting in a combination of these movements.

Q. 51. **Why are saddle joints able to perform a wide range of movements?**
Answer: Saddle joints are able to perform a wide range of movements because of following reasons:
- Their reciprocally saddle-shaped articular surfaces allow complex articulations similar to condyloid joints but with greater freedom.

Q. 52. **Why do ball and socket joints provide the greatest range of movement?**
Answer: Ball and socket joints provide the greatest range of movement because of following reasons:
- Their rounded convex surface fits into a cup-like socket, allowing movements around multiple axes with a common center.

Q. 53. **Why are uniaxial joints restricted to movements in only one plane?**
Answer: Uniaxial joints are restricted to movements in only one plane because of following reasons:
- Their structural design permits motion around a single axis, such as the transverse or vertical axis.

Q. 54. **Why do biaxial joints allow movements in 2 planes?**
Answer: Biaxial joints allow movements in two planes because of following reasons:
- Their structure supports
    - Flexion and extension around one axis and
    - Abduction and adduction around another, enabling a range of complex movements.

Q. 55. **Why do multiaxial joints permit movements in 3 planes?**
Answer: Multiaxial joints permit movements in 3 planes because of following reasons:
- Their ball and socket structure allows
    - Flexion, extension,
    - Abduction, adduction,
    - Rotation, and circumduction, offering extensive mobility.

Q. 56. **Why is the synovial joint structure important for active movements like elevation and depression?**
Answer: The synovial joint structure is important for active movements like elevation and depression because of following reasons:
- It allows for smooth, lubricated motion with minimal friction, facilitating efficient and pain-free movements.

Q. 57. **Why can't accessory movements at synovial joints be performed actively by the patient?**
Answer: Accessory movements at synovial joints can't be performed actively by the patient because of following reasons:
- These slight movements require external force or manipulation to occur, which the body's own muscles cannot produce.

Q. 58. **Why do synovial joints permit movements such as protraction and retraction?**
Answer: Synovial joints permit movements such as protraction and retraction because of following reasons:
- They are designed to allow forward and backward motion of body parts, essential for activities like chewing and speaking.

Q. 59. **Why do sensory nerve endings in the fibrous capsule of synovial joints trigger reflex contraction of muscles?**
Answer: Sensory nerve endings in the fibrous capsule of synovial joints trigger reflex contraction of muscles because of following reasons:
- To protect the joint by positioning it in a manner that maximizes
    - Comfort and
    - Stability,
    - Preventing dislocation.

Q. 60. **Why are active movements like elevation and depression possible at synovial joints?**
Answer: Active movements like elevation and depression are possible at synovial joints because of following reasons:
- These joints are structured to allow diverse and precise movements, facilitated by the joint cavity and synovial fluid, which support smooth motion.

Q. 61. **Why does the periarticular network of arteries supply the capsule, synovial membrane, and epiphysis of synovial joints?**
Answer: The periarticular network of arteries supplies the capsule, synovial membrane, and epiphysis of synovial joints because of following reasons:
- It is formed from the branches of arteries lying in the vicinity of the joint.
- It provides essential nutrients and oxygen to these structures.

Q. 62. **Why is the nerve supply to the capsule important for joint stability?**
Answer: The nerve supply to the capsule is important for joint stability because of following reasons:
- It includes encapsulated nerve endings sensitive to proprioceptive sensations and free nerve endings sensitive to pain.
- It ensures

- That the joint's position and
- Any potential damage are effectively monitored.

Q. 63. Why is it necessary for ligaments to be supplied by pain-sensitive free nerve endings?

Answer: It is necessary for ligaments to be supplied by pain-sensitive free nerve endings because of following reasons:
- Provide immediate feedback on any damage or strain,
- Helping to protect the joint from further injury.

Q. 64. Why does Hilton's law state that the nerves supplying a joint also supply the muscles regulating its movements?

Answer: Hilton's law states that the nerves supplying a joint also supply the muscles regulating its movements because of following reasons:
- It ensures coordinated and efficient control of joint actions.
- This helps maintain stability and prevent injury.

Q. 65. Why does gardner's observation ensure the stability of a joint?

Answer: Gardner's observation ensures the stability of a joint because of following reasons:
- The part of the joint capsule rendered taut by muscle contraction.
- It is supplied by a nerve that innervates the antagonist muscles,
- It provides balanced tension and stability during movements.

Q. 66. Why do the bones play an important role in providing the stability of certain synovial joints?

Answer: The bones play an important role in providing the stability of certain synovial joints because of following reasons:
- Their shapes and the way they fit together,
- Such as the head of the femur fitting into the hip bone socket,
- Create natural stability that reduces the likelihood of dislocation.

Q. 67. Why is muscle tone and strength considered the most important factor in maintaining joint stability?

Answer: Muscle tone and strength is considered the most important factor in maintaining joint stability because of following reasons:
- Strong, toned muscles support the joint structures and control movements,
- Therefore preventing instability and dislocation.

Q. 68. Why is acquired dislocation of the hip joint rare?

Answer: Acquired dislocation of the hip joint is rare because of following reasons:
- Hence the head of the femur is perfectly fitted into the socket of the hip bone
- Providing significant stability.

Q. 69. **Why do the cruciate ligaments within the knee joint provide anteroposterior stability?**

Answer: The cruciate ligaments within the knee joint provide anteroposterior stability because of following reasons:
- Thus they prevent excessive forward and backward movements of the knee,
- Ensuring the joint remains stable during various activities.

Q. 70. **Why does weakening or paralysis of muscles acting on a joint lead to instability and potential dislocation?**

Answer: Weakening or paralysis of muscles acting on a joint leads to instability and potential dislocation because of following reasons:
- For the reason that muscles provide crucial support and control for joint movements, and without their proper function,
- The joint is prone to excessive movement and instability.

Q. 71. **Why the close is packed position of a joint most firm and rigid?**

Answer: The close packed position of a joint is most firm and rigid because of following reasons:
- The articular surfaces are fully congruent, all ligaments are taut,
- And the joint is in a position where it cannot be easily pulled apart.

Q. 72. **Why is the loose packed position of a joint prone to dislocation?**

Answer: The loose packed position of a joint is prone to dislocation because of following reasons:
- The articular surfaces are incongruent and the joint space is freely mobile,
- Making it less stable and more susceptible to displacement.

Q. 73. **Why do the ligaments force the articular surfaces to come together in the close packed position?**

Answer: The ligaments force the articular surfaces to come together in the close packed position because of following reasons:
- To ensure maximum contact and stability, minimizing the risk of dislocation.

Q. 74. **Why is damage to intraarticular structures most likely if dislocation occurs in the close packed position?**

Answer: Damage to intra articular structures is most likely if dislocation occurs in the close packed position because of following reasons:
- The joint is in a maximally congruent and stable state, making any forceful displacement likely to cause internal damage.

Q. 75. **Why do joint positions like close packed and loose packed affect joint stability?**

Answer: Joint positions like close packed and loose packed affect joint stability because of following reasons:
- They indicate how the congruence and mobility of articular surfaces,
- Influenced by ligaments, affect the stability and vulnerability to dislocation.

Q. 76. **Why the joint is functionally considered as one in the close packed position?**

Answer: The joint is functionally considered as one in the close packed position because of following reasons:
- The articular surfaces are fully congruent and maximally stable,
- Behaving as a single unit.

Q. 77. **Why does a joint experience reflex spasm of muscles and referred pain to the overlying skin during joint disease?**

Answer: a joint experience reflex spasm of muscles and referred pain to the overlying skin during joint disease because of following reasons:
- According to ton's law, joints are innervated by nerves that also supply the muscles crossing the joint and the skin over it,
- Leading to reflex spasms and pain to stabilize the joint in a comfortable position.

Q. 78. **Why do the synovial cavities of all carpometacarpal joints intercommunicate except the 1st carpometacarpal joint?**

Answer: The synovial cavities of all carpometacarpal joints intercommunicate except the 1st carpometacarpal joint because of following reasons:
- The 1st carpometacarpal joint is an independent cavity.

Q. 79. **Why are all the carpometacarpal joints plane type of synovial joints except the 1st carpometacarpal joint?**

Answer: All the carpometacarpal joints are plane type of synovial joints except the 1st carpometacarpal joint because of following reasons:
- The 1st carpometacarpal joint is a saddle type of synovial joint.

Q. 80. **Why do all the bones in the lower limb provide attachment to muscle/muscles except the talus, which is devoid of any muscular attachment?**

Answer: The talus is devoid of any muscular attachment because of following reason:
- The primary function of talus is weight-bearing. It transmits forces from the tibia to the foot, allowing for smooth movement at the ankle joint.
- Because talus has unique shape and position within the ankle joint.
- It articulates with the tibia, fibula, calcaneus, and navicular bones.

- It provides stability and facilitating the range of motion needed for walking and running.
- Muscular attachments would interfere with these critical functions.
- It would also limit the talus's ability to move freely within the joint.

Q. 81. **Why is the knee joint the only joint in the lower limb whose cavity is traversed by the tendon of a muscle (tendon of popliteus), despite being intracapsular but extrasynovial?**

Answer: Knee joint the only joint in the lower limb whose cavity is traversed by the tendon of a muscle (tendon of popliteus), despite being intracapsular but extrasynovial because of following reasons:
- The knee joint has the tendon of popliteus traversing its cavity to assist in stabilizing the joint during movement.
- Though the tendon is intracapsular, its extrasynovial location ensures it can perform its mechanical function effectively.

Q. 82. **Why do joints affected by disease often exhibit pain referred to the overlying skin?**

Answer: Joints affected by disease exhibit pain referred to the overlying skin because of following reasons:
- Their articular nerves, which supply both the joint and the overlying skin become irritated.
- This irritation leads to reflex spasms of the surrounding muscles, fixing the joint in a position of greater comfort and causing pain to be felt in the skin above.

Q. 83. **Why are dislocations rare in the close- packed position of a joint?**

Answer: Dislocations are rare in the close- packed position of a joint because of following reasons:
- This position maximizes joint stability. Ligaments are taut, joint surfaces are fully congruent,
- And there is maximum contact area between the joint surfaces, making.

Miscellaneous questions

Q. 84. **Why are joints supported by a variety of soft tissue structures?**

Answer: Joints are supported by a variety of soft tissue structures to provide
- Stability and
- Allow for smooth, controlled movement.
- These structures, such as ligaments, tendons, and cartilage, help to stabilize the joint, absorb shock, and reduce friction.
- They ensure that the bones move in a coordinated and efficient manner while maintaining the integrity of the joint.

Q. 85. **Why discs are usually connected to their fibrous capsule by vascularized connective tissue?**

Answer: Discs are usually connected to their fibrous capsule by vascularized connective tissue because of following reasons:
- They become invaded by
    - Blood vessels and
    - Afferent and vasomotor postganglionic sympathetic nerves.

Q. 86. **Why is the function of intra-articular fibrocartilage uncertain?**

Answer: The function of intra-articular fibrocartilage is uncertain because of following reasons:
1. **Evidence from structural or phylogenetic data**: studies of intra-articular fibrocartilage, such as menisci or articular discs, show structural variations across different species and joints. These variations suggest that the fibrocartilage may serve different roles based on its
    - Location and
    - Evolutionary context.
2. **Aided by mechanical analogies**: mechanical analogies help in understanding the potential functions of fibrocartilage. For example, comparing it to cushioning materials or load-distributing devices highlights its possible role in shock absorption and load distribution.
3. **Multiple potential functions**: the uncertainty stems from the fact that intra-articular fibrocartilage could serve several functions simultaneously or differently in various joints.
4. **Improving fit between articulating surfaces**: intra-articular fibrocartilage often conforms to the shape of the joint surfaces, enhancing the fit and possibly stabilizing the joint.
5. **Deployment of weight over larger surface areas**: by spreading the load over a broader area, fibrocartilage helps reduce stress on the joint surfaces, which is particularly important in weight-bearing joints.
6. **Shock absorption**: the fibrocartilage's ability to compress and deform under pressure provides a shock-absorbing effect, protecting the joint from excessive forces.

These points collectively explain why the function of intra-articular fibrocartilage is considered uncertain and multifaceted.

Q. 87. **Why are fat pads soft and able to change shape to fill joint recesses?**

Answer: Fat pads are soft and able to change shape to fill joint recesses because
- They vary in dimension according to joint position,
- They act as cushion and support the joint.

Q. 88.   **Why are cartilaginous structures within joints normally avascular?**
Answer: Cartilaginous structures within joints are normally avascular because of following reason:
- High mechanical pressures in these deformable tissues would collapse any blood vessels inside them.

Q. 89.   **Why is learning ill-understood greek names not helpful for understanding joints?**

Answer: Learning ill-understood Greek names is not helpful for understanding joints because of following reason:
- These names might not provide meaningful information about
    o   The structure,
    o   Function, or
    o   Location of the joints, making it harder to grasp their significance.
- Instead, focusing on the functional and anatomical aspects of joints can provide a clearer and more practical understanding.

Q. 90.   **Why is a purely structural classification of joints considered the best approach? Ai**
Answer: A purely structural classification of joints is considered the best approach because of following reason:
- It directly reflects their physical characteristics and how they are connected. This classification provides clear information about joint stability and range of motion.

Q. 91.   **Why is the embryological development of synovial joints important to understand their anatomy?**
Answer: Understanding the embryological development of synovial joints is important because of following reason:
- It reveals how these joints form and acquire their structures. This knowledge helps explain their functional characteristics and potential developmental issues.

Q. 92.   **Why are muscles considered indispensable for maintaining stability in most joints?**
Answer: Muscles are considered indispensable for maintaining stability in most joints because of following reasons:
- They prevent excessive movement against sudden stresses,
- Support the joint structures.
- It is specially true in unstable joints like the knee and shoulder.

Q. 93. Why is the skull type of joint classified as immovable?

Answer: The skull type of joint is classified as immovable because of following reasons:
- These joints allow for no movement.
- The articulating bones are joined by tough fibrous tissue, such as the sutures of the skull.
- Which do not permit any significant movement.

Q. 94. Why is the limb type of joint classified as freely movable?

Answer: The limb type of joint is classified as freely movable because of following reasons:
- These joints are synovial joints with a wide range of movement.
- They have a synovial cavity filled with synovial fluid.
- Which allows for various types of movements like flexion, extension, abduction, adduction, and rotation.

Q. 95. Why is a simple joint classified as such?

Answer: A simple joint is classified as such because of following reasons:
- It involves articulation between 2 bones.
- For example, the interphalangeal joints.
- These joints allow movement in one plane.

Q. 96. Why a compound is joint classified as such?

Answer: A compound joint is classified as such because of following reasons:
- It involves articulation between more than 2 bones within one joint capsule.
- Examples include the elbow joint and wrist joint.
- There is articulations of multiple bones.

Q. 97. Why a complex is joint classified as such?

Answer: A complex joint is classified as such because of following reasons:
- Its joint cavity is divided by an intra- articular disc
- Such as in the temporomandibular joint, acromioclavicular joint, and sternoclavicular joint.
- These joints often have complex movements and functions due to the presence of the intra-articular disc.

Q. 98. Why is the anterior fontanelle used to judge the hydration of the infant?

Answer: The anterior fontanelle is used to judge the hydration of the infant because of following reasons:
- It is a reliable indicator of the baby's fluid balance.
- If the fontanelle is sunken, it may indicate dehydration.

Q. 99. **Why are synovial joints categorized as freely movable joints (diarthroses)?**
Answer: Synovial joints are categorized as freely movable joints (diarthroses) because of following reasons:
- They have a synovial cavity filled with fluid, enabling a wide range of motion and flexibility.

Q. 100. **Why are fat pads able to accommodate the changing conditions of a joint?**
Answer: Fat pads are able to accommodate the changing conditions of a joint because of following reasons:
- They are pliant and can adjust to different movements and pressures within the joint.

Q. 101. **Why gliding or slipping movements at synovial joints are considered the simplest type of movement?**
Answer: Gliding or slipping movements at synovial joints are considered the simplest type of movement because of following reasons:
- They involve flat bone surfaces moving past each other in a linear fashion without any significant rotation or angular movement.

Q. 102. **Why is there usually no dislocation in the close packed position of a joint?**
Answer: There is usually no dislocation in the close packed position of a joint because of following reasons:
- The articular surfaces are fully congruent and firmly held together by taut ligaments, preventing separation.

Q. 103. **Why does joint disease lead to reflex spasms of muscles and pain referred to the overlying skin, according to Hilton's law?**
Answer: Joint disease lead to reflex spasms of muscles and pain referred to the overlying skin, according to Hilton's law because of following reason:
- Hilton's law indicates that joints are innervated by nerves that also supply the muscles and skin over the joint, causing reflex reactions during irritation.

Q. 104. **Why do all the bones of the first row of carpals take part in the formation of the wrist joint except the pisiform?**
Answer: All the bones of the first row of carpals take part in the formation of the wrist joint except the pisiform because of following reasons:
- The pisiform does not participate in the wrist joint formation due to its anatomical position and function.

Q. 105. Why are all the joints in the upper limb synovial joints except intermediate radio-ulnar joints?

Answer: All the joints in the upper limb are synovial joints except intermediate radio-ulnar joints because of following reasons:
- Intermediate radio-ulnar joints are fibrous joints (syndesmosis).

Q. 106. Why are all the superficial muscles on the front of the forearm supplied by the median nerve except the flexor carpi ulnaris?

Answer: The flexor carpi ulnaris muscle is supplied by the ulnar nerve instead of the median nerve because of because of following reasons:
- Its embryological development and nerve distribution.
- During development, the muscles in the forearm are divided into different compartments, with the median nerve typically supplying most of the muscles in the anterior compartment.
- However, the flexor carpi ulnaris, along with part of the flexor digitorum profundus, develops in a way that aligns it with the ulnar nerve's pathway, leading to its innervation by the ulnar nerve instead.

Q. 107. Why are all the intrinsic muscles of the hand supplied by the ulnar nerve except the muscles of thenar eminence and lateral two lumbricals?

Answer: The intrinsic muscles of the hand are predominantly supplied by the ulnar nerve because of their development and the nerve distribution pattern.
- However, the muscles of the thenar eminence and the lateral 2 lumbricals are supplied by the median nerve. They are closely associated with the flexor muscles of the forearm, which are mainly innervated by the median nerve.
- This distinct innervation pattern allows for precise and fine motor control of the thumb and index and middle fingers, which are crucial for tasks like gripping and pinching.

Q. 108. Why is the calcaneus the only short bone (either carpals or tarsals) that regularly has an epiphysis, covering its posterior surface and ossifying by a secondary center that appears at different ages in males and females before fusion?

Answer: The calcaneus is the only short bone that regularly has an epiphysis because of following reason:
- It has critical role in weight-bearing and movement.
- The posterior surface of the calcaneus forms the calcaneal tuberosity, where the Achilles tendon attaches, and exerting significant force during activities like walking, running, and jumping.
- To accommodate and distribute these forces effectively, the calcaneus develops a secondary ossification center, which forms an epiphysis that strengthens the bone at this attachment site.
- The secondary ossification center appears at different ages in males and females due to differences

- - In growth rates and
  - The timing of skeletal maturity between genders.
- This process ensures that the calcaneus can continue to develop and strengthen during the years when the demands on the Achilles tendon and calcaneal tuberosity are greatest.

3. Muscle

Skeletal Muscle

Q. 1. Why are muscle forces capable of moving limbs and driving many functions of the human body?

Answer: Muscle forces are capable of moving limbs and driving many functions of the human body because of following reason:
- Muscle tissue, constitutes a significant portion of body mass.
- It is specialized for converting chemical energy into mechanical work.
- It facilitates movement and other physiological processes.

Q. 2. Why do skeletal muscle fibres exhibit cross-striations when viewed microscopically?

Answer: Skeletal muscle fibres exhibit cross-striations when viewed microscopically because of following reason:
- Their myosin and actin filaments are organized into regular, repeating structures called sarcomeres.
- They give the cells a finely cross-striated appearance.

Q. 3. Why are lipid droplets more common in muscle fibres with a high mitochondrial content and good capillary blood supply?

Answer: Lipid droplets are more common in muscle fibres with a high mitochondrial content and good capillary blood supply because of following reason:
- They represent a rich source of energy.
- The energy can be tapped by oxidative metabolic pathways.
- They are prevalent in such fibres.

Q. 4. Why is acetylcholine (ACh) rapidly bound by receptor molecules in the synaptic cleft?

Answer: Acetylcholine (ach) is rapidly bound by receptor molecules in the synaptic cleft because of following reason:
- It triggers instantaneous increase in the permeability.
- It results in conductance, of the postsynaptic membrane.
- It leads to muscle depolarization.

Q. 5. **Why is excitation-contraction coupling essential for muscle contraction?**
Answer: Excitation-contraction coupling is essential for muscle contraction because of following reason:
- It triggers the release of calcium from the sarcoplasmic reticulum into the cytosol.
- This activates a calcium-sensitive switch in the thin filaments.
- It initiates the process of muscle contraction.

Q. 6. **Why do the lengths of thick and thin filaments not change during muscle contraction?**
Answer: The lengths of thick and thin filaments do not change during muscle contraction because of following reason:
- Muscle contraction occurs through the sliding of thick and thin filaments
- They draw the Z-discs towards the middle of each sarcomere.
- It shortens the sarcomere without altering the length of the individual filaments.

Q. 7. **Why is ATP essential for myosin head binding and release during muscle contraction?**
Answer: ATP is essential for myosin head binding and release during muscle contraction because of following reason:
- These processes are energy-dependent.
- ATP is required for myosin heads to bind to actin filaments.
- It acts as power strokes, and release from actin filaments.
- It allows cycling of cross-bridge interactions which is necessary for muscle contraction.

Q. 8. **Why do skeletal muscles work in pairs?**
Answer: Skeletal muscles work in pairs because of following reason:
- They can only pull, not push.
- One muscle (the agonist) contracts to move a joint, while the opposing muscle (the antagonist) relaxes.

Q. 9. **Why skeletal muscles are also called striped muscles?**
Answer: Skeletal muscles are called striped muscles because of following reason:
- Their fibers have a striped appearance under a microscope due to alternating light and dark bands.

Q. 10. **Why do we refer to skeletal muscles as striated muscles?**
Answer: Skeletal muscles are referred to as striated muscles because of following reason:
- Their fibers contain repeating sarcomeres that give them a striped or striated appearance.

Q. 11. **Why the origin of a muscle considered is fixed during its contraction?**
Answer: The origin of a muscle remains fixed during contraction because of following reason:
- It is typically attached to a more stationary bone.

Q. 12. **Why the fleshy part of a muscle is called the "belly"?**
Answer: The fleshy part of a muscle is called the "belly" because of following reason:
- It is the thicker, more contractile part of the muscle.

Q. 13. **Why the fibrous part of a muscle is called a "tendon" when cord-like or rope-like?**
Answer: The fibrous part of a muscle is called a "tendon" when cord-like or rope-like because of following reason:
- It attaches muscle to bone and is not contractile.

Q. 14. **Why is the fibrous part of a muscle called an "aponeurosis" when flattened?**
Answer: The fibrous part of a muscle is called an "aponeurosis" when flattened because of following reason:
- It spreads out like a broad, flat sheet of connective tissue.

Q. 15. **Why are muscle fibres multinucleated?**
Answer: Muscle fibres are multinucleated because of following reason:
- They are formed by the fusion of several myoblasts during development.

Q. 16. **Why are dark bands in myofibrils called a bands?**
Answer: Dark bands in myofibrils are called a bands because of following reason:
- They are anisotropic.

Q. 17.   **Why do most skeletal muscles contain a mixture of fibre types?**
Answer: Most skeletal muscles contain a mixture of fibre types because of following reason:
- Different muscles serve different functions that require varying levels of endurance and strength.

Q. 18.   **Why is the connective tissue in muscles important?**
Answer: The connective tissue in muscles is important because of following reason:
- It provides structural support and organization by surrounding and connecting muscle fibres, fascicles, and the entire muscle.

Q. 19.   **Why are Z discs important in myofibrils?**
Answer: Z discs are important in myofibrils because of following reason:
- They anchor and organize the actin filaments, which are essential for muscle contraction.

Q. 20.   **Why do sarcomeres appear cross-striated?**
Answer: Sarcomeres appear cross-striated because of following reason:
- The alignment of dark A bands and light I bands across myofibrils.

Q. 21.   **Why is the perimysium important in muscles?**
Answer: The perimysium is important in muscles because of following reason:
- It surrounds and supports bundles (fascicles) of muscle fibres, providing additional structural organization.

Q. 22.   **Why do parallel fasciculi muscles have a greater range of movement compared to their oblique counterparts?**
Answer: Parallel fasciculi muscles have a greater range of movement compared to their oblique counterparts because of following reason:
- Their fibers are aligned with the direction of pull.
- They allow longer contractions and greater range of movement.

Q. 23.   **Why are muscles like the biceps and triceps named according to the number of heads of origin?**
Answer: Muscles like the biceps and triceps are named according to the number of heads of origin because of following reason:
- This nomenclature provides a clear description of their anatomical structure.
- It indicates the number of tendinous origins of the muscle.

Q. 24. **Why do muscles like the rectus abdominis have intervening tendons or intersections?**

Answer: Muscles like the rectus abdominis have intervening tendons or intersections because of following reason:
- To provide structural support.
- It allows
  - Greater flexibility and
  - Range of movements.
- It contributes the stability and function of the abdominal wall.

Q. 25. **Why are muscles that extend over 2 or more joints called diarthric or polyarthric muscles?**

Answer: Muscles that extend over two or more joints are called diarthric or polyarthric muscles because of following reason:
- Their actions affect multiple joints.
- They, allow coordinate complex movements across the joints,
- Examples are
  - Biceps brachii,
  - Flexor carpi radialis and
  - Flexor digitorum profundus.

Q. 26. **Why is the size of a motor unit dependent upon the precision of muscle control?**

Answer: The size of a motor unit is dependent upon the precision of muscle control because of following reason:
- Smaller motor units with fewer muscle fibers are required for fine, precise movements.
- Larger motor units with more fibers are sufficient for gross, less precise movements.

Q. 27. **Why do skeletal muscles attach to the skeleton?**

Answer: Skeletal muscles attach to the skeleton because of following reason:
- To facilitate movements and for the stability of the body.
- The attachment of tendons, allow for efficient transmission of force to produce movement.

Q. 28. **Why is the knowledge restricted to skeletal muscles clinically more relevant?**

Answer: The knowledge is restricted to skeletal muscles because of following reason:
- They are voluntary muscles involved in movement. And their injuries, diseases, and conditions are more directly relevant in clinical practice.

Q. 29. **Why are skeletal muscles most abundant in the body?**

Answer: Skeletal muscles are most abundant because of following reason:
- They are located superficially and attached to the skeleton, making them easily accessible for movement and support.

Q. 30. **Why skeletal muscles are commonly displayed during cadaver dissections?**

Answer: Skeletal muscles are commonly displayed during cadaver dissections because of following reason:
- To study their anatomy and function in relation to the skeleton and their role in movement.

Q. 31. **Why are skeletal muscles tested by clinicians in clinical practice, particularly for paralysis and intramuscular injections?**

Answer: Clinicians test skeletal muscles because of following reason:
- They are voluntary and essential for movement, making them critical for assessing paralysis and administering intramuscular injections.

Q. 32. **Why do skeletal muscles perform the function of levers to move the body and its appendages?**

Answer: Skeletal muscles act as levers because of following reason:
- When they contract, they produce movement at joints, enabling activities such as walking, running, and other daily activities.

Q. 33. **Why does metabolism within skeletal muscle cells increase heat production during strenuous exercises?**

Answer: Skeletal muscle cells increase heat production during strenuous exercises because of following reason:
- As a by-product of metabolism, which helps maintain body temperature and supports metabolic processes.

Q. 34. **Why do skeletal muscles maintain posture and body support even when the body is at rest?**
Answer: Skeletal muscles maintain posture and body support even when the body is at rest because of following reason:
- Continuously to stabilize joints and keep the body in an upright position, even during periods of rest.

Q. 35. **Why are synovial bursae and synovial sheaths important in muscle anatomy?**
Answer: Synovial bursae and synovial sheaths are important because of following reason:
- They reduce friction between
    - Tendons and
    - Other structures, allowing for smooth movement.

Q. 36. **Why do synovial bursae form around tendons?**
Answer: Synovial bursae form around tendons because of following reason:
- Tendons rub against
    - Bone,
    - Cartilage,
    - Ligaments, or
    - Other tendons, necessitating a lubricating device to reduce friction.

Smooth Muscle

Q. 37. **Why are single-unit smooth muscles found in the intestines?**
Answer: Single-unit smooth muscles are found in the intestines because of following reason:
- Their structure allows for coordinated contractions through mechanical pull between fused cell membranes
- It facilitates the rhythmic movements necessary for peristalsis and the movement of contents through the digestive tract.

Q. 38. **Why do multi-unit smooth muscles have a rich nerve supply?**
Answer: Multi-unit smooth muscles have a rich nerve supply because of following reason:
- Each muscle cell receives a separate nerve fibre.
- It allows for precise and simultaneous control of muscle contraction, as seen in structures like the ductus deferens.

Q. 39. **Why are myoepithelial cells spindle-shaped?**
Answer: Myoepithelial cells are spindle-shaped because of following reason:
- To facilitate contractions
- It aids in the expulsion of secretions from glands such as salivary and mammary glands.

Q. 40. **Why do smooth muscles form the walls of viscera?**
Answer: Smooth muscles form the walls of viscera because of following reason:
- To enable involuntary movements, such as peristalsis, that are necessary for the function of organs like
    - The intestines,
    - Blood vessels, and
    - Urinary bladder.

Q. 41. **Why do skeletal, cardiac, and smooth muscles share the properties of irritability, contractility, extensibility, and elasticity?**
Answer: Skeletal, cardiac, and smooth muscles share the properties of irritability, contractility, extensibility, and elasticity because of following reason:
- These muscles share these properties because they are essential for their functions:
    - Irritability allows them to respond to stimuli,
    - Contractility enables them to shorten when stimulated,
    - Extensibility lets them return to their original length, and
    - Elasticity allows them to assume their shape after being stretched.

Q. 42. **Why are the structure and functions of smooth muscles better understood when studying the involuntary organs of the body?**
Answer: The structure and functions of smooth muscles are better understood in the context of studying involuntary organs because of following reason:
- Smooth muscles form the walls of these organs and are crucial for their involuntary movements and functions.

Cardiac Muscle

Q. 43. **Why are sympathetic nerves important for the heart?**
Answer: Sympathetic nerves are important for the heart because of following reason:

- They stimulate both the heart rate and blood pressure, and dilate the coronary arteries.
- They are essential for increasing cardiac output and provides adequate blood flow to the heart muscle itself.

Q. 44. Why do parasympathetic fibers decrease the heart rate?
Answer: Parasympathetic fibers decrease the heart rate because of following reason:
- They oppose the actions of the sympathetic nerves.
- It helps to lower heart rate and restore normalcy after periods of stress or exertion.

Q. 45. Why do cardiac muscles form the wall of the heart (myocardium)?
Answer: Cardiac muscles form the myocardium of the heart because of following reason:
- To provide the contractile force needed to pump blood throughout the body.
- It, ensures circulation and oxygenation of tissues.

Q. 46. Why do skeletal, smooth, and cardiac muscles differ considerably from each other?
Answer: Skeletal, smooth, and cardiac muscles differ considerably because of following reason:
- Due to variations in their
    - Structure,
    - Function, and
    - The mechanisms by which they are controlled.
- They, reflect the specialized roles in the body.

Q. 47. Why are the structure and functions of cardiac muscles better understood when studying the heart?
Answer: The structure and functions of cardiac muscles are better understood when studying the heart because of following reason:
- Cardiac muscles form the myocardium and are responsible for the continuous and rhythmic contraction needed to pump blood throughout the body.

General Muscle/Other

Q. 48. **Why do most cells possess cytoskeletal elements capable of lengthening or shortening?**

Answer: Most cells possess cytoskeletal elements capable of lengthening or shortening because of following reason:
- In order to change shape,
- It enables various cellular functions such as
    - Locomotion,
    - Phagocytosis, and mitosis.

Q. 49. **Why are slow movements effected by polymerization-depolymerization mechanisms involving actin and tubulin?**

Answer: Slow movements are effected by polymerization-depolymerization mechanisms involving actin and tubulin because of following reason:
- These mechanisms allow for
    - Controlled and
    - Gradual changes in cell shape, contributing to processes such as cellular locomotion.

Q. 50. **Why can much faster and more forceful movements be created by motor proteins using energy from the hydrolysis of ATP?**

Answer: Much faster and more forceful movements can be created by motor proteins using energy from the hydrolysis of ATP because of following reason:
- ATP-dependent systems provide a more
    - Rapid and
    - Powerful means of generating cellular movement compared to polymerization-depolymerization mechanisms.

Q. 51. **Why has the ability of specialized cells, like muscle cells, to change shape become their most important property?**

Answer: The ability of specialized cells, like muscle cells, to change shape has become their most important property because of following reason
- It enables them to perform essential functions such as contraction.
- It is vital for processes like
    - Locomotion and
    - Driving various functions of the human body.

Q. 52. **Why is the neurovascular hilum significant in muscles?**
Answer: The neurovascular hilum is important in muscles because of following reason:
- It serves as the entry point for major source arteries, veins, and nerves
- It subsequently branch within the muscle's connective tissue framework.

Q. 53. **Why is the classification of muscle vascular anatomy into 5 types relevant?**
Answer: The classification of muscle vascular anatomy into 5 types is relevant because of following reason:
- It helps in determining survival of muscle.
- It is useful for pedicled or free tissue transfer procedures in
  - Plastic and
  - Reconstructive surgery.

Q. 54. **Why do muscles involved in sustained activities have a denser capillary network?**
Answer: Muscles involved in sustained activities have a denser capillary network because of following reason:
- They require more
  - Oxygen and
  - Nutrients for prolonged contraction.
- The denser network ensures efficient delivery of these resources.

Q. 55. **Why do veins and arteries in muscles form territories and anastomose with each other?**
Answer: Veins and arteries in muscles form territories and anastomose with each other because of following reason:
- To ensure continuous blood supply even if one route is compromised.
- Thus it
  - Maintains adequate perfusion and
  - Prevents ischemia.

Q. 56. **Why do vessels tend not to cross between muscles?**
Answer: Vessels tend not to cross between muscles because of following reason:
- There is relative movement within muscle groups.
- They radiate to muscles from more stable sites.
- They cross at points of fusion.
- This is to maintain stability and prevent damage.

Q. 57. **Why is the concept of angiosomes important in understanding muscle vascularization?**
Answer: The concept of angiosomes is important because of following reason:
- It helps to understand the composite blocks of tissues.
- It is supplied by specific distributing arteries and drained by their companion veins.
- It provides understanding of the vascular territories and their clinical relevance.

Q. 58. **Why does pressure exerted on valved intramuscular veins during muscle contraction promote venous return to the heart?**
Answer: Pressure exerted on valved intramuscular veins during muscle contraction promotes venous return to the heart because of following reason:
- It acts as a "muscle pump".
- It enhances
  - The efficiency of blood circulation and
  - Prevents venous stasis.

Q. 59. **Why do nerves travel through the epimysial and perimysial septa before entering the endomysial tissue around muscle fibers?**
Answer: Nerves travel through the epimysial and perimysial septa before entering the endomysial tissue around muscle fibers because of following reason:
- To reach their target muscle fibers efficiently.
- It helps to coordinate muscle contraction and sensory feedback.

Q. 60. **Why the neuromuscular junction is considered a specialized synapse?**
Answer: The neuromuscular junction is considered a specialized synapse because of following reason:
- It facilitates communication between motor neurons and muscle fibers.
- It allows
  - The transmission of action potentials and
  - Subsequent muscle contraction.

Q. 61. **Why is fibre type transformation significant in muscle adaptation?**
Answer: Fibre type transformation is significant in muscle adaptation because of following reason:
- It allows muscles to adjust their contractile and metabolic properties in response to changing physiological demands or stimuli.
- This transformation helps to optimise muscle function.
- It performs under different conditions.

Q. 62. **Why does grouping of fibres with similar properties occur after nerve damage?**

Answer: Grouping of fibres with similar properties occurs after nerve damage because of following reason:
- Denervated fibres may be 'taken over' by sprouting motor neurons.
- It leads to the adoption of similar metabolic and contractile properties.
- This process helps to maintain muscle function despite nerve damage.

Q. 63. **Why do fast muscles develop slow contractile characteristics after continuous stimulation?**

Answer: Fast muscles develop slow contractile characteristics after continuous stimulation because of following reason:
- The pattern of impulse traffic in the nerves innervates the muscles.
- It influences fibre type transformation.
- Continuous stimulation at a slower frequency induces changes in muscle properties, leading to slower contraction and increased resistance to fatigue.

Q. 64. **Why is reversibility of fibre type transformation important?**

Answer: The reversibility of fibre type transformation is important because of following reason:
- It demonstrates that changes in muscle properties occur within existing fibres rather than through degeneration and regeneration.
- This reversibility allows muscles to adapt dynamically to changing physiological conditions.

Q. 65. **Why do myoblasts become spindle-shaped and express muscle-specific proteins during muscle development?**

Answer: Myoblasts become spindle-shaped and express muscle-specific proteins during muscle development because of following reason:
- They undergo differentiation and preparation for fusion to form multinucleate cylindrical syncytia, or myotubes.
- They are the building blocks of skeletal muscle fibers.

Q. 66. **Why is the initiation of fusion of myoblasts important for sarcomere formation?**
Answer: The initiation of fusion of myoblasts is important for sarcomere formation because of following reason:
- The synthesis of the contractile machinery is not dependent on fusion.
- The sarcomere formation proceeds more rapidly after fusion.
- It, leads to
    - The assembly of myofibrils and
    - The development of muscle structure and function.

Q. 67. **Why do myofibrils continue to add sarcomeres to their ends during muscle development?**
Answer: Myofibrils continue to add sarcomeres to their ends during muscle development because of following reason:
- To increase muscle fiber length. This process allows for the optimization of mean sarcomere length and filament overlap.
- They are essential for maximizing muscle force generation.

Q. 68. **Why do satellite cells play a crucial role in muscle repair and regeneration?**
Answer: Satellite cells play a crucial role in muscle repair and regeneration because of following reason:
- They have the capability to proliferate and differentiate into myoblasts.
- They can fuse with damaged muscle fibers or form new myotubes.
- This process replenishes damaged muscle tissue and promotes its recovery after injury.

Q. 69. **Why is muscle mass regulation important for muscle adaptation?**
Answer: Muscle mass regulation is important for muscle adaptation because of following reason:
- Muscles respond to various stimuli such as
    - Resistance exercise or
    - Inactivity by undergoing hypertrophy (increased mass) or
    - Atrophy (decreased mass).
- These adaptations help optimize muscle function and performance in different physiological conditions.

Q. 70. **Why are muscles classified into 3 types based on morphological and functional characteristics?**
Answer: Muscles are classified into skeletal, smooth, and cardiac types because of following reason:

- Each type has distinct structures and functions adapted to their respective roles in the body.

Miscellaneous questions

Q. 71. Why are the names given to individual muscles usually descriptive and based on various characteristics such as shape, size, number of heads or bellies, position, depth, attachments, or actions?

Answer: The names given to individual muscles are usually descriptive and based on various characteristics because of following reason:
- They provide information about the morphology, location, and functional roles of the muscles X.
- They aid in identification and understanding of the roles in movement and support.

Q. 72. Why should the functional roles implied by the names of muscles be interpreted with caution?

Answer: The functional roles implied by the names of muscles should be interpreted with caution because of following reason:
- They are often oversimplified.
- The terms may denote one of the several actions.
- A given muscle may play different roles in different movements.
- These roles may change depending on various factors such as assisted or opposed movements by gravity.

Q. 73. Why do muscles exhibit different fiber architectures?

Answer: Muscles exhibit different fiber architectures because of following reason:
- They need to accommodate varying functional demands such as
  - Generating force,
  - Moving tendons through a considerable distance, or
  - Maintaining stability.
- Different fiber architectures allow muscles to optimize their performance in different physiological contexts.

Q. 74. **Why is the resultant force of a muscle directed along the line of the tendon?**

Answer: The resultant force of a muscle is directed along the line of the tendon because of following reason:
- Muscles generate tension along their fibers, and the tendon serves as a structural connection between the muscle and the bone it moves.
- Therefore, the force exerted by the muscle is transmitted along the tendon to produce movement at the attachment site.

Q. 75. **Why do powerful muscles tend to be long as well as fat?**

Answer: Powerful muscles tend to be long as well as fat because of following reason:
- Power, which is the rate at which a muscle can perform external work, depends on both
    - Force and
    - Contraction velocity.
- Longer muscles can accommodate more muscle fibers, increasing the total force-generating capacity.
- The fat muscles can generate more force due to a larger cross-sectional area.

Q. 76. **Why does the author argue against naming epimysia?**

Answer: The author argues against naming epimysia because of following reason:
- They believe it complicates descriptive anatomy unnecessarily and perplexes students.

Q. 77. **Why do muscles with oblique fibers fall into different patterns?**

Answer: Muscles with oblique fibers fall into different patterns because of following reason:
- Variations in their tendon formations and
- The arrangement of muscle fibers.

Q. 78. **Why is it important for clinicians to have detailed knowledge of the surface appearances of muscles?**

Answer: It is important for clinicians to have detailed knowledge of the surface appearances of muscles because of following reason:
- It aids in diagnosis, especially in distinguishing between different types of pain or tenderness.

Q. 79. **Why are muscle origins and insertions described as having no reality?**
Answer: Muscle origins and insertions are described as having no reality because of following reason:
- Their fixed and moving ends depend on
  - Circumstances and
  - Vary with most muscles.

Q. 80. **Why do fleshy origins generally leave no mark on the bone?**
Answer: Fleshy origins generally leave no mark on the bone because of following reason:
- They may flatten or depress the area without leaving a distinct mark.

Q. 81. **Why do flat muscles that arise from flat bones have a characteristic origin pattern?**
Answer: Flat muscles that arise from flat bones have a characteristic origin pattern because of following reason:
- Their origin extends to a curved line set back from the bone's edge.
- It allows a greater range of movement.

Q. 82. **Why is it difficult to have objective proof of the primary action of most muscles?**
Answer: It is difficult to have objective proof of the primary action of most muscles because of following reason:
- Common sense is often needed to assess the results, and various methods of study have limitations.

Q. 83. **Why is the action of paradox important in clinical investigations of muscle function?**
Answer: The action of paradox is important in clinical investigations of muscle function because of following reason:
- It involves a reversal of muscular action against gravity, which must be considered in understanding certain movements.

Q. 84. **Why do muscles have a rich blood supply?**
Answer: Muscles have a rich blood supply because of following reason:
- To provide oxygen and nutrients necessary for their function.
- To remove metabolic waste products.

Q. 85. **Why does the name "muscles" come from the Latin word "mus"?**
Answer: The name "muscles" come from the Latin word "mus" because of following reason:
- The name "muscles" comes from the Latin word "mus" because "mus" means "mouse."

Q. 86. **Why are smooth muscles important in the body?**
Answer: Smooth muscles are important because of following reason:
- They regulate the movement of substances through hollow organs (like the digestive tract) and blood vessels.
- They, help in the process of digestion and circulation.

Q. 87. **Why do slow muscle fibres appear red in colour?**
Answer: Slow muscle fibres appear red in colour because of following reason:
- They contain large amounts of myoglobin.

Q. 88. **Why are fast muscle fibres easily fatigued?**
Answer: Fast muscle fibres are easily fatigued because of following reason:
- They rely on glycolytic respiration, which is less efficient in generating energy compared to aerobic metabolism.

Q. 89. **Why are slow muscle fibres highly resistant to fatigue?**
Answer: Slow muscle fibres are highly resistant to fatigue because of following reason:
- They have a well-developed aerobic metabolism, with abundant mitochondria and oxidative enzymes.

Q. 90. **Why do oblique fasciculi arrangements result in more powerful muscles?**

Answer: Oblique fasciculi arrangements result in more powerful muscles because of following reason:
- The oblique orientation allows a greater number of muscle fibers to attach to the tendon.
- Thereby increases the force that the muscle can generate.

Q. 91. **Why might a muscle with a multipennate fasciculi arrangement be stronger but have a limited range of motion?**

Answer: A muscle with a multipennate fasciculi arrangement might be stronger but have a limited range of motion because of following reason:
- The oblique orientation of the fibers increases the force generation capacity.
- It results in a reduction in the length of fiber contraction.
- And thus, a limited range of motion.

Q. 92. **Why are spiral or twisted fasciculi advantageous in muscles like the trapezius and pectoralis major?**

Answer: Spiral or twisted fasciculi are advantageous in muscles like the trapezius and pectoralis major because of following reason:
- They allow these muscles to perform complex, multidirectional movements.
- Hence increase the functional versatility.

Q. 93. **Why are the range of movements in strap-like muscles with tendinous intersections maximized?**

Answer: The range of movements in strap-like muscles with tendinous intersections is maximized because of following reason:
- The structure allows these muscles to stretch and contract along the entire length of the muscle.
- Thus they facilitate extensive movement.

Q. 94. **Why do muscles with circumpennate fasciculi have increased strength at the cost of movement range?**

Answer: Muscles with circumpennate fasciculi have increased strength at the cost of movement range because of following reason:
- The radial arrangement of fibers around a central tendon increases the cross-sectional area.
- Hence enhances production of force but limits the length of fibre and thus, decreases range of movement.

Q. 95. **Why do the different arrangements of muscle fasciculi indicate specific functional capabilities of the muscles?**

Answer: The different arrangements of muscle fasciculi indicate specific functional capabilities of the muscles because of following reason:
- The orientation and organization of fibers determine both
    - The generation of force and
    - Range of motion that the muscle can achieve.

Q. 96. **Why is the reason for the increased power in pennate muscles associated with their fiber arrangement?**

Answer: The reason for the increased power in pennate muscles is associated with their fiber arrangement because of following reason:
- The angled fibers allow more fibers to pack into a given muscle volume.
- Thus it increases the total force of the muscle.

Q. 97. **Why do bipennate muscles have a reduced range of motion compared to unipennate muscles?**

Answer: Bipennate muscles have a reduced range of motion compared to unipennate muscles because of following reason:
- The arrangement of fibers on both sides of the tendon shortens the effective fiber length.
- It limits the extent of contraction.

Q. 98. **Why are cruciate muscles like the sternocleidomastoid able to perform complex movements?**

Answer: Cruciate muscles like the sternocleidomastoid are able to perform complex movements because of following reason:
- Their crossed fasciculi arrangement allows them to act in multiple directions and contribute to various types of movements.

Q. 99. **Why do multipennate muscles, such as the deltoid, exhibit greater strength?**

Answer: Multipennate muscles, such as the deltoid, exhibit greater strength because of following reason:
- The multiple tendons have higher density of muscle fibers.
- It enhances the overall force of the muscle.

Q. 100. **Why are muscle spindles important for proprioception?**

Answer: Muscle spindles are important for proprioception because of following reason:
- They act as stretch receptors that detect changes in muscle length and tension.
- It provides feedback to the central nervous system to help regulate and coordinate muscle contractions and maintain posture and balance.

Q. 101. **Why is the sensory function of parasympathetic fibers important?**
Answer: The sensory function of parasympathetic fibers is important because of following reason:
- They are involved in visceral reflexes.
- They convey painful impulses from the heart, which are crucial for maintaining homeostasis and responding to potential cardiac issues.

Q. 102. **Why does the length of fleshy fibers affect the range of movement?**
Answer: The length of fleshy fibers affects the range of movement because of following reason:
- It determines how much the muscle can contract and shorten during isotonic contraction.
- It directly influences the amplitude of movement.

Q. 103. **Why are fixators important in muscle function?**
Answer: Fixators are important in muscle function because of following reason:
- They stabilize the proximal joints of a limb.
- They allow the distal joints to perform movement on a stable base. ,
- This is essential for precise and controlled movements.

Q. 104. **Why are synergists necessary for movements involving multiple joints?**
Answer: Synergists are necessary for movements involving multiple joints because of following reason:
- They prevent undesired actions at the proximal joints while the prime movers perform the desired action.
- It, ensures coordination and efficiency in movement.

Q. 105. **Why do sympathetic nerves dilate the coronary arteries?**
Answer: Sympathetic nerves dilate the coronary arteries because of following reason:
- To increase blood flow to the heart muscle during periods of increased activity or stress.
- It ensures that the heart receives adequate oxygen and nutrients.

Q. 106. **Why is isotonic contraction important for muscle function?**
Answer: Isotonic contraction is important for muscle function because of following reason:
- It allows the muscle to change its length.
- It moves a body part, facilitates movements such as walking, running, and lifting.

Q. 107. **Why do antagonists help prime movers by controlled relaxation?**
Answer: Antagonists help prime movers by controlled relaxation because of following reason:
- To ensure smooth and precise movements.
- This controlled relaxation prevents excessive or unwanted movements and allows the prime movers to perform their actions effectively.

Q. 108. **Why are synergists important for making a tight fist?**
Answer: Synergists are important for making a tight fist because of following reason:
- They stabilize the wrist joint in extension while the long digital flexors contract to flex the fingers.
- It, ensures that the wrist remains stable and allows for precise finger movements.

Q. 109. **Why are muscles classified and named according to their function?**
Answer: Muscles are classified and named according to their function because of following reason:
- To describe their roles in movement and to facilitate understanding of their actions in various anatomical contexts.
- It helps in clinical diagnosis and planning of treatment.

Q. 110. **Why are myofibroblasts important in wound healing?**
Answer: Myofibroblasts play a crucial role in wound healing because of following reason:
- Due to their ability to contract, which helps in closing wounds and remodeling the tissue during the healing process.

Q. 111. **Why are skeletal muscles described in detail compared to other muscle types?**
Answer: Skeletal muscles are described in detail because of following reason:
- They are clinically more relevant due to their involvement in movement, posture, and common injuries, especially in athletes.

Q. 112. **Why are subtendinous bursae the most common type in the limbs?**
Answer: Subtendinous bursae are common because of following reason:
- They intervene between
  - Tendon and bone,
  - Ligament, or
  - Between two tendons, reducing friction during movement.

Q. 113. **Why do tendons passing through fibrous bands have synovial sheaths?**
Answer: Tendons passing through fibrous bands have synovial because of following reason:
- Sheaths to reduce friction and provide a lubricating environment, enabling smooth movement.

Q. 114. **Why are neuromuscular spindles crucial in muscle function?**
Answer: Neuromuscular spindles crucial in muscle function because of following reason:
- They provide sensory information to
    - Control muscle tone and
    - Participate in the stretch reflex,
    - Helping to maintain posture and
    - Coordinate movement.

Q. 115. **Why do muscles have different types of contractions?**
Answer: Muscles have different types of contractions because of following reason:
- Isometric contractions maintain muscle length while increasing tension.
- Isotonic contractions change muscle length while maintaining tension, enabling varied movements.

Q. 116. **Why is the segmental innervation of muscles important?**
Answer: The segmental innervation of muscles is important because of following reason:
- It helps understand which spinal segments control which muscles.
- It aids in clinical evaluation and treatment of neuromuscular disorders.

Q. 117. **Why are innervation impulses distributed equally to the extra-ocular muscles of each eye?**
Answer: Innervation impulses distributed equally to the extra-ocular muscles of each eye because of following reason:
- Ton's Law states that this equal distribution provides an explanation for the secondary deviation of the sound eye when one or more muscles are paralyzed in the other eye.

Q. 118. **Why are innervation impulses equally distributed to the extra-ocular muscles of each eye, according to Hering's Law?**
Answer: Innervation impulses equally distributed to the extra-ocular muscles of each eye, according to Hering's Law because of following reason:
- Hering's Law states that this equal distribution explains the secondary deviation of the sound eye when muscles are paralyzed in the other eye.

Q. 119. **Why does joint disease lead to reflex spasms of muscles and pain referred to the overlying skin, according to Hilton's Law?**
Answer: Joint disease lead to reflex spasms of muscles and pain referred to the overlying skin, according to Hilton's Law because of following reason:
- Hilton's Law indicates that nerve supplying the muscles acting on the joint supplies
    o Joint and
    o Skin over joint.

Q. 120. **Why are all intrinsic muscles of the larynx supplied by the recurrent laryngeal nerve, except cricothyroid?**
Answer: All intrinsic muscles of the larynx supplied by the recurrent laryngeal nerve, except cricothyroid because of following reason:
- Embryological explanation:
    o Cricothyroid develops from fourth pharyngeal arch and nerve of the fourth pharyngeal arch is external laryngeal nerve.
    o All the muscles of the larynx except cricothyroid are developed from 6th pharyngeal arch and the nerve of the sixth pharyngeal arch is recurrent laryngeal nerve.
- Physiological (functional correlation): The cricothyroid muscle acts as a tuning fork. First, it receives impulses and starts vibrating. The remaining muscles receive impulses few milli-second afterwards, which help in producing voice.

Q. 121. **Why are all the extra-ocular muscles of the eye supplied by the 3rd cranial nerve, except lateral rectus and superior oblique? AI**
Answer: All the extra-ocular muscles of the eye supplied by the 3rd cranial nerve, except lateral rectus and superior oblique because of following reason:
- Lateral rectus is supplied by the 6th cranial nerve and superior oblique by the 4th cranial nerve, illustrating the specialized innervation of these eye muscles.

Q. 122. **Why are all the intrinsic muscles of the larynx paired, except inter-arytenoid (transverse arytenoid)? AI**

Answer: All the intrinsic muscles of the larynx paired, except inter-arytenoid (transverse arytenoid) because of following reason:
- Inter-arytenoid (transverse arytenoid) is unpaired, indicating an exception to the general pattern of paired muscles in the larynx.

Q. 123. **Why are all the muscles on the front of the arm attached to the humerus except the biceps brachii?**

Answer: All the muscles on the front of the arm attached to the humerus except the biceps brachii because of following reason:
- The biceps brachii attaches to the scapula above and the radius below.

Q. 124. **Why is the brachioradialis the only long muscle in the body attached to the distal ends of two long bones? AI**

Answer: The brachioradialis the only long muscle in the body attached to the distal ends of two long bones because of following reason:
- It attaches to the distal ends of the humerus and radius.

Q. 125. **Why are all the superficial muscles on the front of the forearm supplied by the median nerve except the flexor carpi ulnaris? AI**

Answer: All the superficial muscles on the front of the forearm supplied by the median nerve except the flexor carpi ulnaris because of following reason:
- The flexor carpi ulnaris is supplied by the ulnar nerve.

Q. 126. **Why are all the intrinsic muscles of the hand supplied by the ulnar nerve except the muscles of the thenar eminence and the lateral two lumbricals? AI**

Answer: All the intrinsic muscles of the hand supplied by the ulnar nerve except the muscles of the thenar eminence and the lateral two lumbricals because of following reason:
- The muscles of the thenar eminence and the lateral 2 lumbricals are supplied by the median nerve.

Q. 127.   **Why is pronator quadratus the only muscle in the body attached to the distal ends of two long bones lying parallel to each other? AI**

Answer: Pronator quadratus the only muscle in the body attached to the distal ends of two long bones lying parallel to each other because of following reason:
- It attaches to the distal ends of the radius and ulna.

Q. 128.   **Why do all the bones in the upper limb provide attachment to muscle or muscles except the lunate and triquetral bones?**

Answer: All the bones in the upper limb provide attachment to muscle or muscles except the lunate and triquetral bones because of following reason: AI
- The lunate and triquetral bones are devoid of muscular attachments, serving primarily as structural components of the wrist.

Q. 129.   **Why are all the superficial muscles on the front of the forearm supplied by the median nerve except the flexor carpi ulnaris? AI**

Answer: All the superficial muscles on the front of the forearm supplied by the median nerve except the flexor carpi ulnaris because of following reason:
- The flexor carpi ulnaris is supplied by the ulnar nerve.

Q. 130.   **Why are all the intrinsic muscles of the hand supplied by the ulnar nerve except the muscles of thenar eminence and lateral two lumbricals? AI**

Answer: All the intrinsic muscles of the hand are supplied by the ulnar nerve except the muscles of thenar eminence and lateral two lumbricals because of following reason:
- These muscles are supplied by the median nerve.

Q. 131.   **Why do all the bones in the lower limb provide attachment to muscle/muscles except the talus, which is devoid of any muscular attachment?**

Answer: Bones in the lower limb provide attachments to muscles to facilitate movement and stability, but the talus lacks muscular attachments because of following reason:
- To maintain its structural role in transmitting weight and supporting the ankle joint.

Q. 132. **Why do the external intercostal muscles in the 10th and 11th intercostal spaces extend forwards up to the tips of the costal cartilages, whereas all the other external intercostal muscles do not extend beyond the junction of ribs with their costal cartilages?**

Answer: The external intercostal muscles in the 10th and 11th intercostal spaces extend forwards up to the tips of the costal cartilages because of following reason:
- To provide additional support and mobility to the lower ribs during respiratory movements, ensuring flexibility and proper expansion of the thoracic cage during breathing.

4. Lymphatic system

Lymphatic system and immunity

Q. 1. Why is the lymphatic system crucial for providing immunological defenses?

Answer: The lymphatic system is crucial for providing immunological defenses because of following reason:
- It transports and filters lymph, which contains white blood cells, especially lymphocytes.
- These cells detect and respond to pathogens.
- They help in fighting the infections.
- Additionally, lymph nodes act as sites where immune responses are initiated.

  It enables the lymphatic system to protect the body against diseases.

Q. 2. Why are lymph nodes essential in the lymphatic system's role in immunity?

Answer: Lymph nodes are essential in the lymphatic system's role in immunity because of following reason:
- They
  - Filter lymph,
  - Capturing and destroying pathogens, and
  - They house immune cells that respond to infections.

Q. 3. Why do lymph nodes enlarge during infections?

Answer: Lymph nodes enlarge during infections because of following reason:
- They are actively filtering out pathogens.
- They produce more immune cells to fight the infection.

Q. 4. Why does lymph from the small intestine appear milky white?

Answer: Lymph from the small intestine is milky white because of following reason:
- Known as chyle, because it contains large fat droplets absorbed from the intestine.

Q. 5. **Why do lymph nodes evoke an immunological response?**
Answer: Lymph nodes evoke an immunological response because of following reason:
- They produce antibodies in response to infection.
- They, help activate lymphocytes.
- They serve as sites for
    - The production and
    - Maturation of various types of lymphocytes.

Q. 6. **Why are cells of the reticulo-endothelial system involved in phagocytosis?**
Answer: Cells of the reticulo-endothelial system are involved in phagocytosis because of following reason:
- They play a crucial role in the body's defense mechanism.
- These cells, including macrophages, are specialized in engulfing and digesting foreign particles, bacteria, and dead cells.
- Phagocytosis helps clear harmful substances from the body, aiding in immune response and tissue maintenance.

Q. 7. **Why are lymphocytes crucial in the immune response?**
Answer: Lymphocytes are crucial in the immune response because of following reason:
- They are specialized cells that circulate in the blood and lymphatic organs.
- They are capable of recognizing and responding to specific antigens.
- Thus they provide a targeted defense against pathogens.

Q. 8. **Why are T lymphocytes named as such?**
Answer: T lymphocytes are named because of following reason:
- They mature and undergo processing in the thymus gland.
- It is essential for their development and differentiation into various types of T cells.
- They provide cell-mediated immunity.

Q. 9. **Why are B lymphocytes named after the bursa of Fabricius?**
Answer: B lymphocytes are named after the bursa of Fabricius because of following reason:
- A cloacal diverticulum in birds, because it was first discovered in chickens that this structure plays a key role in the
    - Maturation and
    - Differentiation of b cells.
- These are responsible for antibody-mediated (humoral) immunity in mammals.

Q. 10. **Why do cytotoxic T lymphocytes, helper T lymphocytes, and memory T lymphocytes play different roles in the immune response?**
Answer: Cytotoxic T lymphocytes, helper T lymphocytes, and memory T lymphocytes play different roles in the immune response because of following reason:
- They are specialized T cells that respond to antigens in distinct ways:
- Cytotoxic T cells destroy infected cells,
- Helper T cells support other immune cells, and
- Memory T cells provide long-term immunity.

Q. 11. **Why are plasma cells and memory B lymphocytes functionally distinct?**
Answer: Plasma cells and memory B lymphocytes are functionally distinct because of following reason:
- Plasma cells produce and release antibodies (immunoglobulins) that bind to antigens and neutralize them.
- Memory B cells provide long-lasting immunity by remembering how to quickly produce specific antibodies upon subsequent exposure to the same antigen.

Q. 12. **Why is the thymus important in the differentiation of T-lymphocytes?**
Answer: The thymus is important in the differentiation of T-lymphocytes because of following reason:
- It helps immature T-cells become immunologically competent and capable of recognizing and responding to a wide range of foreign antigens.

Q. 13. **Why do lymphocytes pass through different zones in the cortex of a lymph node?**

Answer: Lymphocytes pass through different zones in the cortex of a lymph node because of following reason:
- To mature and differentiate.
- They move from the germinal center (zone 3) to the outer zone (zone 1) and then to the lymph sinus, supported by macrophages.

Q. 14. **Why the Mononuclear Phagocyte System is closely related to the lymphatic system?**

Answer: The Mononuclear Phagocyte System (Reticulo-endothelial System) is closely related to the lymphatic system because of following reason:
- Both are independent structurally and functionally.
- The system consists of highly phagocytic cells distributed throughout the body, including macrophages and monocytes, which play a key role in immune responses and clearing cellular debris.

Q. 15. **Why do lymph capillaries absorb large protein molecules and particulate matter from tissue spaces?**

Answer: Lymph capillaries absorb large protein molecules and particulate matter from tissue spaces because of following reason:
- To remove cellular debris and foreign particles, such as dust particles inhaled into the lungs, bacteria, and other microorganisms.
- These are then conveyed to regional lymph nodes.

Q. 16. **Why do lymph nodes act as filters for lymph and prevent foreign particles from entering the bloodstream?**

Answer: Lymph nodes act as filters for lymph and prevent foreign particles from entering the bloodstream because of following reason:
- By percolating lymph slowly through their intricate network of spaces.
- This allows macrophages in the sinuses to engulf foreign particles and trap antigens.

Q. 17. **Why are mature B-lymphocytes (plasma cells) and T-lymphocytes produced in lymph nodes?**
Answer: Mature B-lymphocytes (plasma cells capable of producing antibodies) and T-lymphocytes are produced in lymph nodes because of following reason:
- To mount both cellular and humoral immune responses against antigen-laden phagocytes.

Q. 18. **Why is the production and maturation of B- and T-lymphocytes the main function of lymphoid tissue?**
Answer: The production (proliferation) and maturation of B- and T-lymphocytes is the main function of lymphoid tissue because of following reason:
- To ensure an effective immune response against pathogens and foreign particles encountered in the body.

Q. 19. **Why are Malpighian corpuscles important in the spleen?**
Answer: Malpighian corpuscles important in the spleen because of following reason:
- They form part of the white pulp in the spleen.
- It consists of lymphatic sheaths and nodules that are crucial for the spleen's immunological functions.

Lymphatic system and fluid balance

Q. 20. **Why does the lymphatic system act as a drainage system for excess tissue fluid?**
Answer: The lymphatic system acts as a drainage system for excess tissue fluid because of following reason:
- It collects and returns this fluid, known as lymph, back into the bloodstream.
- This helps maintain fluid balance in the body and prevents tissue swelling.

Q. 21. **Why is the lymphatic system essential for fluid balance in the body?**
Answer: The lymphatic system is essential for fluid balance in the body because of following reason:
- It collects excess tissue fluid and returns it to the bloodstream.
- It prevents edema and maintains proper circulation.

Q. 22. **Why is the tissue fluid that enters the lymph capillaries called lymph?**
Answer: The tissue fluid entering lymph capillaries is termed lymph because of following reason:
- It contains
    - Proteins,
    - Fats, and
    - Other particles.
- These substances are similar to plasma but lacks plasma proteins.

Q. 23. **Does lymph carry away larger particles like bacteria and cell debris?**
Answer: Lymph carries away larger particles like bacteria and cell debris because of following reason:
- To filter and destroy them in the lymph nodes.
- It prevents entering into circulation of the body.

Q. 24. **Why is the constitution of lymph similar to that of plasma to some extent?**
Answer: The constitution of lymph is similar to that of plasma because of following reason:
- It contains
    - Lymphocytes,
    - Macromolecules of protein,
    - Fat droplets, and
    - Particulate matter.
- It lacks plasma proteins.

Q. 25. **Why do smaller lymph vessels merge to form larger lymph ducts?**
Answer: Smaller lymph vessels merge to form larger lymph ducts because of following reason:
- To efficiently transport lymph towards the subclavian veins where it re-enters the circulatory system.

Q. 26. **Why does the thoracic duct drain lymph from most of the body except the right upper quadrant?**
Answer: The embryological basis for the drainage pattern of the thoracic duct and right lymphatic duct because of following reason:
- Lies in the development of the lymphatic system.

- During embryogenesis, the lymphatic system develops from 6 primary lymph sacs.
- The thoracic duct originates from the cisterna chyli, a lymph sac in the abdominal region. The connection of these sacs forms the thoracic duct. It grows and ascends along the developing spine.
- As the embryo develops, lymphatic vessels from the left side of
- The body, and most of the lower body, connect with the thoracic duct.
- The right lymphatic duct, however, develops separately to drain the right upper quadrant.
- It includes
    - The right side of the head,
    - Neck,
    - Chest, and
    - Right arm.
- This separation reflects the embryological division of the lymphatic drainage regions, which persists into adulthood.

Q. 27. **Why are lymphatic vessels able to transport lymph against gravity?**
Answer: Lymphatic vessels are able to transport lymph against gravity because of following reason:
- Due to the contraction of smooth muscle in their walls, pulsation of nearby arteries, massaging action from surrounding muscles, and the presence of valves that prevent backflow.

Q. 28. **Why is most of the tissue fluid formed at the arterial end of capillaries absorbed back into the blood by the venous ends of the capillaries and postcapillary venules?**
Answer: Most of the tissue fluid formed at the arterial end of capillaries is absorbed back into the blood by the venous ends of the capillaries and postcapillary venules because of following reason:
- The osmotic pressure difference and reabsorption mechanisms in these vessels.

Lymphatic vessels and capillaries

Q. 29. **Why do lymph capillaries begin blindly in the tissue spaces?**
Answer: Lymph capillaries begin blindly in the tissue spaces because of following reason:
- They need to efficiently absorb excess tissue fluid that cannot be reabsorbed by the venous ends of capillaries.

Q. 30.   **Why are the walls of lymph capillaries more permeable to tissue fluid containing large molecules?**

Answer: The walls of lymph capillaries are more permeable to tissue fluid containing large molecules because of following reason:
- To facilitate
    - The absorption of proteins,
    - Particulate matter, and
    - Colloidal material from the intercellular spaces.

Q. 31.   **Why do lymph capillaries differ from blood capillaries?**

Answer: Lymph capillaries differ from blood capillaries because of following reason:
- They begin blindly in intercellular spaces.
- They have a larger and less regular lumen.
- They are permeable to larger molecules.

Q. 32.   **Why are lymph capillaries absent in certain sites such as the epidermis and brain?**

Answer: Lymph capillaries are absent in certain sites like the epidermis and brain because of following reason:
- These areas have alternative mechanisms for fluid drainage and immune defense.
- The epidermis relies on blood capillaries for nutrient exchange.
- the brain uses
    - The blood-brain barrier and
    - Cerebrospinal fluid to manage fluid balance and protect against pathogens.

Q. 33.   **Why are lymph capillaries absent in structures like hair and nails?**

Answer: Lymph capillaries are absent in structures like hair and nails because of following reason:
- These structures are made of dead cells.
- They do not require a blood supply or lymphatic drainage.
- They are non-living tissues, so they do not participate in fluid exchange or immune functions.

Q. 34. **Why do lymphatic vessels have a beaded appearance?**
Answer: Lymphatic vessels have a beaded appearance because of following reason:
- They have valves at regular intervals along the vessels.
- These valves prevent the back flow of lymph.
- These valve causes slight bulge in wall and, create a beaded look.

Q. 35. **Why is the flow of lymph in lymphatic vessels unidirectional?**
Answer: The flow of lymph in lymphatic vessels is unidirectional because of following reason:
- There is presence of one-way valves that prevent the back flow of lymph.
- These valves ensure that lymph moves in a single direction, from the tissues towards the heart
- It facilitates proper fluid drainage and immune function.

Q. 36. **Why do lymphatic vessels pass through a series of lymph nodes before draining into the venous system?**
Answer: Lymphatic vessels pass through a series of lymph nodes because of following reason:
- To filter the lymph and remove
    - Pathogens and
    - Harmful agents before it is drained into the venous system.

Q. 37. **Why do lymphatic ducts have valves in their lumen?**
Answer: Lymphatic ducts have valves in their lumen because of following reason:
- To prevent
    - Backflow of lymph and
    - To ensure unidirectional flow towards the subclavian veins.

Q. 38. **Why are superficial lymph vessels found in the superficial fascia deep to the skin?**
Answer: Superficial lymph vessels are found in the superficial fascia deep to the skin because of following reason:
- This location allows them to efficiently collect lymph from the skin and subcutaneous tissues.
- The superficial fascia is a layer of connective tissue that lies just beneath the skin and contains

- o Fat,
- o Blood vessels, and
- o Lymph vessels.
- By being located here, superficial lymph vessels can easily capture
  - o Excess interstitial fluid,
  - o Waste products, and
  - o Immune cells from the skin and nearby tissues, transporting them to deeper lymph nodes for filtration and immune response.
- This strategic placement is crucial for maintaining fluid balance and defending against infections in the skin and superficial tissues.

Q. 39. **Why are deep lymph vessels found deep to the deep fascia and accompany the blood vessels?**

Answer: Deep lymph vessels are found deep to the deep fascia and accompany blood vessels because of following reason:
- They are responsible for draining lymph from the deeper tissues, including
  - o Muscles,
  - o Bones, and
  - o Internal organs.
- These deeper tissues produce lymph as a result of metabolic activities and need an efficient way to transport this lymph to lymph nodes. It ultimately reaches into the bloodstream.
- By accompanying blood vessels, deep lymph vessels can effectively follow the same pathways as the arteries and veins, ensuring that lymph from the deeper regions is efficiently collected and transported.
- This close association with blood vessels also allows the deep lymphatic system to take advantage of the pressure changes from nearby arteries and muscles, which helps to propel the lymph through the vessels.
- This anatomical arrangement ensures proper drainage of lymph from the body's deeper structures.

Q. 40. **Why do lymphatics anastomose freely with their neighbors of the same side as well as of the opposite side?**

Answer: Lymphatics anastomose freely with their neighbors of the same side as well as of the opposite side because of following reason:
- To provide alternative routes for lymphatic drainage, ensuring efficient removal of tissue fluid and particulate matter.

Q. 41.   **Why are the thoracic duct and right lymphatic duct important in the lymphatic system?**

Answer: The thoracic duct and right lymphatic duct are important in the lymphatic system because of following reason:
- They are the main channels through which lymph is returned to the bloodstream.
- The thoracic duct collects lymph from most of the body and drains it into the left subclavian vein,
- The right lymphatic duct drains lymph from the right side of the head, neck, chest, and right arm into the right subclavian vein.
- This process is essential for maintaining fluid balance and allowing the immune system to filter and fight infections.

Q. 42.   **Why do lymphatics have vasa vasorum and a plexus of fine blood vessels?**

Answer: Lymphatics have vasa vasorum and a plexus of fine blood vessels because of following reason:
- To supply nutrients and oxygen to their walls. Lymphatic vessels, especially larger ones, have thick walls that need their own blood supply to maintain their structure and function.
- The vasa vasorum and fine blood vessels ensure that these lymphatic vessels stay healthy and can effectively transport lymph throughout the body.

Lymphoid organs and tissues

Q. 43.   **Why does cancer of the tongue have the worst prognosis if located in the posterior third of the tongue?**

Answer: The posterior third of the tongue because of following reason:
- Has a rich lymphatic drainage and
- Proximity to vital structures, leading to early spread and a worse prognosis.

Q. 44. **Why is lymphatic spread the most common route of spread of cancer of the tongue?**
Answer: Lymphatic spread the most common route of spread of cancer of the tongue Cancer of the tongue because of following reason:
- Commonly spreads through the lymphatics due to the extensive lymphatic network in the oral cavity.

Lymphatic system and development

Q. 45. **Why does the lymphoid tissue of the body grow rapidly during childhood and cease growth around puberty?**
Answer: The lymphoid tissue of the body grows rapidly during childhood and ceases growth around puberty because of following reason:
- Due to its role in immune function and development.
- This growth pattern is shared by
    - Lymph nodes,
    - Thymus,
    - Tonsils,
    - Lymphoid tissue of the intestines, and
    - Spleen follicles.

Lymphatic system and immunity

Q. 46. **Why do mature lymphocytes join the circulating pool of lymphocytes?**
Answer: Mature lymphocytes join the circulating pool of lymphocytes because of following reason:
- To be readily available to respond to antigenic emergencies, contributing to the body's immune defense mechanisms.

Q. 47. **Why the bone marrow is considered a part of the lymphatic system?**
Answer: Bone marrow is considered a part of the lymphatic system because of following reason:
- It produces lymphocytes, which are essential cells of the immune system.
- These lymphocytes, including b cells and t cells, play a key role in identifying and fighting off infections
- It makes bone marrow integral part of the body's immune defenses.

Miscellaneous questions

Q. 48. **Why Haemal nodes are considered an intermediate stage between a lymph node and the spleen?**

Answer: Haemal nodes are considered an intermediate stage between a lymph node and the spleen because of following reason:
- They resemble lymph nodes in structure, but their sinuses are filled with blood rather than lymph. In humans, the spleen is considered a large haemal node.

Q. 49. **Why the thoracic duct is considered the largest lymphatic channel in the body?**

Answer: The thoracic duct is considered the largest lymphatic channel in the body because of following reason:
- It drains lymph from most of the body into the venous system.

Q. 50. **Why the cisterna chyli is considered the largest lymphatic sac in the body?**

Answer: The cisterna chyli is considered the largest lymphatic sac in the body because of following reason:
- It is a major collecting vessel for lymph from the lower body before it enters the thoracic duct.

Q. 51. **Why is Muller's gland important in male anatomy?**

Answer: Muller's gland, or the lymph node in the femoral canal, is important because of following reason:
- It drains the glans penis, indicating its role in the lymphatic drainage of the genitalia.

Q. 52. **Why are Peyer's nodules significant in immunology?**

Answer: Peyer's nodules, or solitary lymphatic follicles, are significant because of following reason:
- They play a role in the immune response in the gut, indicating their importance in protecting against intestinal pathogens.

Q. 53. **Why are Peyer's patches clinically relevant in gastrointestinal pathology?**

Answer: Peyer's patches are clinically relevant because of following reason:
- They are aggregations of lymphatic follicles in the small intestine that become ulcerated in typhoid fever, indicating their role in immune surveillance and in the pathology of gastrointestinal infections.

Q. 54. **Why is the absorption of fat from the intestine an important function of the lymphatic system?**

Answer: The absorption of fat from the intestine is an important function of the lymphatic system because of following reason:
- It allows dietary fats to enter the bloodstream, where they can be transported to tissues for energy and storage.

Q. 55. **Why do lymphocytes develop from pluripotent stem cells in red bone marrow?**

Answer: Lymphocytes develop from pluripotent stem cells in red bone marrow because of following reason:
- This is where they originate and differentiate into mature lymphocytes.
- They are then transported via the bloodstream.
- . They rich various lymphoid tissues where they become immunocompetent.

Q. 56. **Why the lymphatic system is considered accessory to the venous system?**

Answer: The lymphatic system is considered accessory to the venous system because of following reason:
- It functions to drain excess tissue fluid and large particles from the interstitial spaces back into the bloodstream.

Q. 57.   Why is the lymphatic system regarded as a 'drainage system of coarse type'?

Answer: The lymphatic system is regarded as a 'drainage system of coarse type' because of following reason:
- It can remove larger particles, such as
    - Proteins and
    - Particulate matter, from the tissue fluid.
- These particles are not absorbed by the fine drainage system of the venous system.

Q. 58.   Why are certain parts of the lymphatic system (lymph-reticular organs) involved in phagocytosis and raising immune responses?

Answer: Certain parts of the lymphatic system (lympho-reticular organs) are involved in phagocytosis and raising immune responses because of following reason:
- They contain lymphocytes and phagocytic cells.
- They help in removing pathogens and foreign particles from the lymph.

Q. 59.   Why are B-lymphocytes differentiated in bone marrow?

Answer: B-lymphocytes are differentiated in bone marrow because of following reason:
- It provides a specialized environment with the necessary signals for their development.
- The bone marrow contains
    - Stromal cells,
    - Growth factors, and
    - Cytokines that guide the maturation of b-lymphocytes from hematopoietic stem cells.
- This environment ensures that
    - B-lymphocytes develop properly,
    - Acquiring the ability to produce antibodies and
    - Play a key role in the adaptive immune response.

Q. 60.   Why do mature lymphocytes join the circulating pool of lymphocytes?

Answer: Mature lymphocytes join the circulating pool of lymphocytes because of following reason:
- To be readily available to respond to antigenic emergencies, contributing to the body's immune defense mechanisms.

Q. 61. **Why lymph nodes are considered small nodules of lymphoid tissue?**
Answer: Lymph nodes are considered small nodules of lymphoid tissue because of following reason:
- They are oval or reniform in shape, ranging from 1-25 mm long, and are found along the course of smaller lymphatics.

Q. 62. **Why is the hilum of a lymph node important?**
Answer: The hilum of a lymph node is important because of following reason:
- It is a slight depression where the artery enters the node and the vein with efferent lymphatics exits.
- Afferent lymphatics enter the node at different parts of its periphery.

Q. 63. **Why are B-lymphocytes found mainly in the medulla of a lymph node?**
Answer: B-lymphocytes found mainly in the medulla of a lymph node because of following reason:
- B-lymphocytes, particularly mature ones (plasma cells), are found mainly in the medulla of a lymph node because this area supports antibody production and response to pathogens.

Q. 64. **Why are blood channels important in the structure of a lymph node?**
Answer: Blood channels are important in the structure of a lymph node because of following reason:
- They provide the necessary blood supply for the node's metabolic needs and support the immune response functions within the node.

Q. 65. **Why do lymph nodes commonly enlarge in response to inflammation or tumor formation?**
Answer: Lymph nodes commonly enlarge in response to inflammation (lymphadenitis) or tumor formation (such as Hodgkin's disease, lymph sarcoma, etc.) because of following reason:
- Due to increased immune activity and the presence of metastatic malignant growths.

5. Cardiovascular system

Smooth muscle and cardiovascular system

Q. 1. Why is smooth muscle referred to as involuntary muscle?
Answer: Smooth muscle is referred to as involuntary muscle because of following reason:
- Its activity is neither initiated nor monitored consciously.

Q. 2. Why is smooth muscle much more variable in form and function compared to striated or cardiac muscle?
Answer: Smooth muscle is much more variable in form and function compared to striated or cardiac muscle because of following reason:
- It has varied roles in different systems of the body,
    - Regulating diameter,
    - Propelling liquids or solids, or
    - Expelling contents in various organs and tissues.

Q. 3. Why is the membrane of smooth muscle cells important for mechanotransduction in small blood vessels?
Answer: The membrane of smooth muscle cells important for mechanotransduction in small blood vessels because of following reason:
- It contains molecules such as
    - Proteoglycans,
    - Glycoproteins, and
    - Glycolipids, forms a thin, negatively charged network called the glycocalyx.
- This glycocalyx is important for mechanotransduction in small blood vessels

    *. **Mechanotransduction** is the process by which cells convert mechanical stimuli into biochemical signals. This process allows cells to respond to changes in their physical environment, such as pressure, stretch, or shear stress. It plays a critical role in various physiological functions, including muscle contraction, bone remodelling, and the regulation of blood flow. Mechanotransduction involves various cellular components, such as ion channels, integrins, and the cytoskeleton, which help transmit mechanical forces into the cell and initiate signaling pathways that lead to specific cellular responses.

Q. 4. **Why are gap junctions important in smooth muscle?**

Answer: Gap junctions important in smooth muscle because of following reasons:
- Gap junctions in smooth muscle provide a low-resistance channel through which electrical excitation and small molecules can pass, enabling a coordinated wave of contraction.
- They are structurally similar to those in cardiac muscle and facilitate rhythmic (phasic) activity in certain types of smooth muscle.

Q. 5. **Why are smooth muscles innervated by unmyelinated axons with cell located in autonomic ganglia?**

Answer: Smooth muscles innervated by unmyelinated axons with cell bodies located in autonomic ganglia muscle because of following reason:
- These axons spread extensively over a large area of muscle, sending branches into muscle fasciculi, and release neurotransmitters at varicosities along their terminals, allowing for widespread control of muscle activity.
- Smooth muscles are innervated by unmyelinated axons with cell bodies located in autonomic ganglia because they are controlled by the autonomic nervous system (ANS), which regulates involuntary bodily functions like
    - Digestion,
    - Blood vessel constriction, and
    - Gland secretion.
- The use of unmyelinated axons in this system allows for
    - A slower,
    - More gradual transmission of signals. This is suitable for the sustained and less rapid responses typical of smooth muscle activity.
- The cell bodies of these neurons are located in autonomic ganglia, which are clusters of nerve cells that serve as relay points for transmitting signals from the central nervous system (CNS) to the target organs.
- This organization allows for the regulation of smooth muscle activity by the sympathetic and parasympathetic divisions of the ANS, ensuring proper control of involuntary bodily functions.

Q. 6. **Why the cytoplasm of a smooth muscle cell is effectively divided into 2 structural domains?**

Answer: The cytoplasm of a smooth muscle cell is effectively divided into 2 structural domains because of following reason:
- To maintain the spindle-like form of the cell and provide an internal scaffold for interactions with other elements.
- This structural organization contributes to the contractile function of smooth muscle.

Q. 7. **Why is electromechanical coupling more commonly seen in unitary and phasic smooth muscles?**

Answer: Electromechanical coupling is more commonly seen in unitary and phasic smooth muscles because of following reason:
- Electrical excitation can be transmitted from cell to cell via gap junctions, allowing for coordinated contraction.

Q. 8. **Why is the regulation of contraction of smooth muscle largely calcium-dependent?**

Answer: The regulation of contraction of smooth muscle is largely calcium-dependent because of following reason:
- An elevation of intracellular calcium levels mediates the activation of myosin. Which initiates the myosin-actin atpase cycle, leading to muscle contraction.
- The regulation of contraction in smooth muscle is largely calcium-dependent because calcium ions (Ca^{2+}) play a central role in initiating the contraction process. When smooth muscle is stimulated, Ca^{2+} enters the cell from the extracellular space. It is also released from intracellular stores within the sarcoplasmic reticulum.
- Once inside the cell, Ca^{2+} binds to a protein called **calmodulin**, forming a Ca^{2+}-calmodulin complex. This complex then activates an enzyme called **myosin light chain kinase** (MLCK). MLCK phosphorylates the myosin light chains, which enables the myosin heads to bind to actin filaments, leading to muscle contraction.
- The level of Ca^{2+} in the cell determines the extent of activation of this pathway, making calcium a key regulator of smooth muscle contraction.
- When Ca^{2+} levels decrease, the contraction process is reversed, and the muscle relaxes. This calcium-dependent mechanism allows smooth muscle to respond appropriately to various physiological stimuli, such as
    - Changes in blood pressure or
    - The need for digestive motility.

Q. 9. **Why does inhibition of myosin phosphatase increase calcium sensitivity in smooth muscle contraction?**

Answer: Inhibition of myosin phosphatase increases calcium sensitivity in smooth muscle contraction because of following reason:
- Inhibition of myosin phosphatase increases calcium sensitivity in smooth muscle contraction because it prevents the dephosphorylation of myosin light chains, which is a critical step in muscle relaxation.
- Normally, after myosin light chains are phosphorylated by myosin light chain kinase (MLCK), they allow myosin to interact with actin, leading to muscle contraction.
- Myosin phosphatase reverses this process by dephosphorylating the myosin light chains, resulting in muscle relaxation.

- When myosin phosphatase is inhibited, the dephosphorylation of myosin light chains is reduced or prevented. This means that even at lower calcium levels, more myosin remains in the phosphorylated, active state, allowing for sustained muscle contraction. As a result, the smooth muscle becomes more sensitive to calcium, because less calcium is needed to maintain contraction. This increased calcium sensitivity is important in regulating the force of contraction in response to various stimuli.

Q. 10. Why is smooth muscle capable of adapting to changing needs and stimuli throughout life?

Answer: Smooth muscle is capable of adapting to changing needs and stimuli throughout life because of following reason:
- Its significant plasticity, allows it to divide and change phenotype. This is in response to various stimuli, such as
  - During pregnancy or
  - In disease conditions.

Q. 11. Why is smooth muscle activation important in arteries and arterioles?

Answer: Smooth muscle activation is important in arteries and arterioles because of following reason:
- It reduces the calibre of the vessel lumen, and thus regulates blood flow,
- It also increases the rigidity of the vessel wall, and affects compliance and elasticity.

Cardiovascular System – General

Q. 12. Why is the cardiovascular system essential for the body?

Answer: The cardiovascular system is essential because of following reason:
- It transports
  Oxygen,
  Nutrients,
  Hormones, and
  Waste products to and from cells.
- It also helps regulate body temperature and maintain fluid balance.
- Without it, cells would not receive the necessary substances for survival, and waste products would not be effectively removed.

Q. 13. Why do arteries decrease in diameter as they extend from the heart?

Answer: Arteries decrease in diameter as they extend from the heart because of following reason:
- Arteries decrease in diameter as they extend from the heart because they branch into smaller arteries and arterioles.
- This branching system helps
  - To distribute blood more efficiently to various tissues and organs.

- To regulate blood flow to peripheral tissues.
- To regulate blood pressure throughout the body.
- To increase the total surface area for fluid exchange.

Q. 14. Why is blood flow faster near the heart compared to the periphery?

Answer: Blood flow is faster near the heart compared to the periphery because of following reason:
- The cross-sectional area of arteries at the heart's exit is larger. It, leads to decrease in velocity as blood moves towards smaller arterioles and capillaries.
- As blood moves into smaller arteries and arterioles further from the heart, the total cross-sectional area increases, which slows the flow rate. This slower flow rate allows for better nutrient and gas exchange at the capillary level.

Q. 15. Why do capillaries have a thin wall?

Answer: Capillaries have a thin wall because of following reason:
- To facilitate the exchange of
  - Nutrients,
  - Gases, and
  - Waste products between the blood and surrounding tissues.

Q. 16. Why is the endothelial barrier important in capillaries?

Answer: The endothelial barrier in capillaries is important because of following reason:
- It regulates the exchange of substances between the blood and interstitial fluid, maintaining homeostasis and tissue function.

Q. 17. Why do arterioles act as precapillary sphincters?

Answer: Arterioles act as precapillary sphincters because of following reason:
- To regulate blood flow into the capillary beds.
- To control the distribution of
  - Nutrients and
  - Oxygen to tissues based on metabolic demands.

Q. 18. Why do venules lack muscle in their walls?

Answer: Venules lack muscle in their walls because of following reason:
- To maintain high permeability.
- To allow for easy exchange of fluids and cells between the blood and surrounding tissues.

Q. 19. Why the cardiovascular system is considered the transport system of the body?

Answer: The cardiovascular system is considered the transport system of the body because of following reason:
- It conveys nutrients to where they are needed.

- It carries away waste products to be expelled.
- It ensures that essential substances reach tissues and organs and that waste is removed efficiently.

Q. 20. **Why is blood referred to as the conveying medium in the cardiovascular system?**
Answer: Blood is referred to as the conveying medium in the cardiovascular system because of following reason:
- It flows in tubular channels (blood vessels) and transports nutrients and waste products throughout the body.

Q. 21. **Why is the heart described as a four-chambered muscular organ?**
Answer: The heart is described as a four-chambered muscular organ because of following reason:
- It has two atria (receiving chambers) and two ventricles (pumping chambers)
- They work together to pump blood to various parts of the body.

Q. 22. **Why arteries are called distributing channels?**
Answer: Arteries are called distributing channels because of following reason:
- They carry blood away from the heart to different parts of the body.

Q. 23. **Why are veins described as draining channels?**
Answer: Veins are described as draining channels because of following reason:
- They carry blood from different parts of the body back to the heart.

Q. 24. **Why are capillaries described as exchange vessels?**
Answer: Capillaries are described as exchange vessels because of following reason:
- They facilitate the exchange of nutrients and metabolites between the blood and tissue fluid.

Q. 25. **Why are blood vessels classified into five functional groups?**
Answer: Blood vessels are classified into five functional groups because of following reason:
- Based on their roles in
    - Distributing blood,
    - Regulating resistance, and
    - Facilitating exchange, acting as
    - Reservoirs, and
    - Providing shunts.
- Blood vessels are classified into five functional groups because each group has a specific role in the circulatory system. These groups are:

- **Arteries**: Carry oxygenated blood away from the heart to the body.
- **Arterioles**: Regulate blood flow and pressure as blood moves from arteries to capillaries.
- **Capillaries**: Facilitate the exchange of oxygen, nutrients, and waste between blood and tissues.
- **Venules**: Collect blood from capillaries and begin the return journey to the heart.
- **Veins**: Return deoxygenated blood back to the heart.

This classification helps in understanding how blood is distributed and regulated throughout the body.

Q. 26. Why does blood flow from the left ventricle to the right atrium in systemic circulation?

Answer: Blood flows from the left ventricle to the right atrium in systemic circulation because of following reason:
- It has circulated through various parts of the body, delivering oxygen and nutrients, and picking up waste products, before returning to the heart.

Q. 27. Why does blood flow from the right ventricle to the left atrium in pulmonary circulation?

Answer: Blood flows from the right ventricle to the left atrium in pulmonary circulation because of following reason:
- It has passed through the lungs where it picks up oxygen and releases carbon dioxide.
- Then returns to the heart to be pumped to the rest of the body.

Q. 28. Why is the regulation of blood pressure crucial for the cardiovascular system?

Answer: The regulation of blood pressure crucial for the cardiovascular system because of following reason:
- It ensures that blood is efficiently circulated throughout the body.
- It provides adequate perfusion to tissues and organs.

Q. 29. Why does the blood in the cardiovascular system serve as a medium for transportation?

Answer: The blood serves as a medium for transportation because of following reason:
- It carries various agents such as
  - Nutrients,
  - Oxygen, and
  - Carbon dioxide, facilitating their delivery and removal from tissues.

Q. 30. **Why do blood vessels need to carry blood to all tissues of the body?**
Answer: Blood vessels need to carry blood to all tissues because of following reason:
- Tissues require a continuous supply of nutrients and oxygen.
- It need to remove waste products to maintain cellular function and overall health.

Q. 31. **Why is the cardiovascular system important for nutrient transport?**
Answer: The cardiovascular system is important for nutrient transport because of following reason:
- It delivers essential nutrients to different parts of the body.
- It ensures proper cellular function and overall health.

Q. 32. **Why does the cardiovascular system remove waste products from organs and tissues?**
Answer: The cardiovascular system removes waste products because of following reason:
- Metabolic processes produce by products that need to be eliminated to prevent toxicity and maintain homeostasis.

Q. 33. **Why is the cardiovascular system crucial for gaseous exchange in the lungs?**
Answer: The cardiovascular system is crucial for gaseous exchange because of following reason:
- It facilitates the intake of oxygen (O_2).
- It helps the elimination of carbon dioxide (CO_2).
- These are vital for cellular respiration and energy production.

Q. 34. **Why does the cardiovascular system carry hormones and other regulatory molecules to target tissues?**
Answer: The cardiovascular system carries hormones and regulatory molecules because of following reason:
- Cardiovascular system carries substances to distant target tissues.
- These substances carry various physiological processes and maintain body functions.

Q. 35. Why does the cardiovascular system help protect the body from infection?

Answer: The cardiovascular system helps protect the body from infection because of following reason:
- It transports leukocytes and their products to sites of infection and injury.
- They are essential components of the immune response.

Q. 36. Why is the cardiovascular system necessary for maintaining homeostasis?

Answer: The cardiovascular system is necessary for maintaining homeostasis because of following reason:
- It ensures the continuous transport of nutrients, gases, hormones, and waste products.
- They are essential for the body's internal balance and overall health.

Q. 37. Why is blood essential in the cardiovascular system?

Answer: Blood is essential in the cardiovascular system because of following reason:
- It serves as the medium for transporting
    - Nutrients,
    - Gases,
    - Hormones, and
    - Waste products throughout the body.

Q. 38. Why does the heart play a crucial role in the cardiovascular system?

Answer: The heart plays a crucial role in the cardiovascular system because of following reason:
- It pumps blood, providing the force necessary for blood to circulate through the blood vessels

Q. 39. Why are blood vessels important in the cardiovascular system?

Answer: Blood vessels are important in the cardiovascular system because of following reason:
- They act as the channel that carry blood to and from different parts of the body.
- They ensure that tissues receive nutrients and oxygen.
- They also ensures the waste products are removed.

Q. 40. Why is the synthesis of plasma proteins in the liver significant for blood function?

Answer: The synthesis of plasma proteins in the liver is significant for blood function because of following reason:

- The following proteins, are synthesised in liver.
    - Albumins,
    - Globulins, and
    - Fibrinogen.
- They maintain following things.
    - Blood viscosity,
    - Immune responses, and
    - Clotting processes.

Cardiovascular System - Arteries and Veins

Q. 41. Why do arteries contain more smooth muscle as they branch?
Answer: Arteries contain more smooth muscle as they branch because of following reason:
- To regulate blood flow and maintain blood pressure.

Q. 42. Why are the minute branches of arteries called arterioles?
Answer: The minute branches of arteries are called arterioles because of following reason:
- They are small vessels that lead to capillaries and control blood flow into tissues.

Q. 43. Why are veins thin-walled?
Answer: Veins are thin-walled because of following reason:
- Their muscular and elastic tissue content is much less than that of arteries.
- This is directly related to the low venous pressure.

Q. 44. Why is the lumen of veins larger than that of the accompanying arteries?
Answer: The lumen of veins is larger than that of the accompanying arteries because of following reason:
- Veins have
    - Thinner walls and
    - Less muscular and elastic tissue content.
    - This allows for a larger lumen.

Q. 45.   **Why do veins have valves?**

Answer: Veins have valves because of following reason:
- They help prevent the back flow of blood.
- They ensure that blood flows in one direction toward the heart.
- This is especially important in the lower parts of the body, where blood must travel against gravity to return to the heart.
- The venous pressure is low (7 mm Hg).

Q. 46.   **Why are valves absent in certain veins?**

Answer: Valves are absent in veins because of following reason:
- Valves are absent in
    - Central veins and
    - Larger veins.
    - Diameter less than 2 mm diameter.
- The absence of valves in these veins is due to
    - The low pressure of blood flow in these veins.
    - There is no necessity of veins.
    - Being close to heart. This reduces the likelihood of back flow.
- In specific veins such as
    - The venae cavae,
    - Hepatic,
    - Renal,
    - Uterine,
    - Ovarian,
    - Cerebral,
    - Spinal,
    - Pulmonary, and
    - Umbilical veins. These veins either
        - Do not need valves due to their size or
        - Have other mechanisms for blood flow regulation.

Q. 47.   **Why do larger veins have nutrient vessels called vasa vasorum?**

Answer: Larger veins have nutrient vessels called vasa vasorum because of following reason:
- Larger veins have vasa vasorum because these vessels supply nutrients to the venous walls, similar to arteries.

Q. 48.   **Why do vasa vasorum vessels penetrate up to the intima in veins?**

Answer: Vasa vasorum vessels penetrate up to the intima in veins probably because of following reason:
- The low venous pressure and low oxygen tension.

Q. 49. **Why are there fewer nerves in veins compared to arteries?**
Answer: There are fewer nerves in veins compared to arteries because of following reason:
- Possibly because veins do not require as much neural control as arteries do.

Q. 50. **Why are arteries in the heart, brain, small intestine, kidneys, and lower limbs commonly narrowed by atheroma?**
Answer: Arteries in the heart, brain, small intestine, kidneys, and lower limbs are commonly narrowed by atheroma because of following reason:
- These areas are particularly susceptible to the accumulation of cholesterol and lipid compounds.
- Accumulation leads to the development of patchy changes in the arterial walls.

Q. 51. **Why are coronary arteries blocked sometimes treated with stents or grafts?**
Answer: Blocked coronary arteries are sometimes treated with stents or grafts because of following reason:
- It helps to open up the blocked area and restore blood flow to the heart muscle.
- It prevents heart attacks and other complications.

Q. 52. **Why does an aneurysm pose a serious risk to health?**
Answer: An aneurysm poses a serious risk to health because of following reason:
- The weakened and thinner wall of the blood vessel can burst.
- It can lead to
    - Severe bleeding and
    - Potentially life-threatening conditions.

Q. 53. **Why do veins have larger lumens compared to arteries?**
Answer: Veins have larger lumens compared to arteries because of following reason:
- They need to accommodate a larger volume of blood.
- The blood returning to the heart is at lower pressure.

Q. 54. **Why venous pressure is generally low compared to arterial pressure?**
Answer: Venous pressure is generally low compared to arterial pressure because of following reason:
- Veins carry blood back to the heart from the capillaries.
- The blood has already lost most of its pressure from the arterial system.

Cardiovascular system - capillaries and microcirculation

Q. 55. Why are capillaries replaced by sinusoids in certain organs like the liver and spleen?

Answer: Capillaries are replaced by sinusoids in certain organs like the liver and spleen because of following reason:
- To accommodate slower blood flow.
- They allow for more extensive exchange between blood and tissue.

Q. 56. Why is the average diameter of a capillary 6-8 microns?

Answer: The average diameter of a capillary is 6-8 microns because of following reason:
- To permit red blood cells to pass through in single file,
- Ensuring efficient exchange of gases and nutrients between blood and tissues.

Q. 57. Why does the size of capillaries vary from organ to organ?

Answer: The size of capillaries varies from organ to organ because of following reason:
- It is smallest in organs like
  - The brain and
  - Intestines (where tight regulation of exchange is critical).
- It is largest (up to 20 microns) in organs like
  - The skin and
  - Bone marrow, where higher blood flow and exchange are needed.

Q. 58. Why are fenestrated capillaries found in renal glomeruli, intestinal mucosa, endocrine glands, and pancreas?

Answer: Fenestrated capillaries are found in renal glomeruli, intestinal mucosa, endocrine glands, and pancreas because of following reason:
- They allow the passage of larger molecules (up to 20-100 microns in size) across their walls.
- Facilitating the filtration and exchange of larger substances like proteins and hormones.

Q. 59. Why do capillary beds and postcapillary venules form an enormous area for exchange between blood and interstitial fluid?

Answer: Capillary beds and postcapillary venules form an enormous area for exchange between blood and interstitial fluid because of following reason:
- To facilitate the exchange of
  - Nutrients,
  - Gases,
  - Metabolites, and
  - Water, ensuring proper cellular function and homeostasis.

Q. 60. Why do capillaries allow migration of leukocytes out of the vessels?
Answer: Capillaries allow migration of leukocytes out of the vessels because of following reason:
- To facilitate
    - The immune response and
    - Inflammation, aiding in defence against pathogens and tissue repair.

Q. 61. Why is the lumen of sinusoids wider (up to 30 microns) and irregular?
Answer: The lumen of sinusoids is wider (up to 30 microns) and irregular because of following reason:
- To allow for the slow passage of blood.
- To accommodate
    - Large cells and
    - Proteins in organs like
        - The spleen,
        - Bone marrow, and
        - Liver.

Q. 62. Why are the walls of sinusoids thinner and sometimes incomplete?
Answer: The walls of sinusoids are thinner and sometimes incomplete because of following reason:
- They are lined by endothelium with phagocytic cells (macrophages).
- They facilitate the exchange of materials between blood and tissue.

Cardiovascular system - lymphatics and anastomoses

Q. 63. Why does excess interstitial fluid from peripheral tissues return to the blood vascular system?
Answer: Excess interstitial fluid returns to the blood vascular system because of following reason:
- It is collected by lymphatic vessels.
- These vessels drain the fluid into larger lymphatic ducts.
- They ultimately empty into the venous system.
- This process helps
    - Maintain fluid balance in the body and
    - Prevents tissue swelling.

Q. 64. **Why the lymphatic system is considered a parallel circulatory system?**
Answer: The lymphatic system is considered a parallel circulatory system because of following reason:
- It collects excess interstitial fluid and returns it to the blood vascular system.
- It maintains fluid balance.
- It aids in immune function.

Q. 65. **Why do arteriovenous anastomoses occur in certain parts of the body?**
Answer: Arteriovenous anastomoses occur in certain parts of the body because of following reason:
- They serve as direct connections between smaller arteries and veins.
- They bypass the capillary bed under certain conditions.

Q. 66. **Why are anastomoses between adjacent angiosomes significant in plastic and reconstructive surgery?**
Answer: Anastomoses between adjacent angiosomes are significant in plastic and reconstructive surgery because of following reason:
- They provide crucial vascular connections for
    - Designing,
    - Evaluating, and
    - Raising axial flaps.
- They enhance the viability of transplanted or reconstructed tissues by ensuring a reliable blood supply.
- This is very much true if the primary blood vessels are damaged or inadequate.
- This helps improve healing and reduces the risk of tissue necrosis.

Q. 67. **Why venous anastomosis is considered communication between veins or their tributaries?**
Answer: Venous anastomosis is considered communication between veins or their tributaries because of following reason:
- It allows for alternate pathways for venous blood flow, such as the dorsal venous arches of the hand and foot.

Q. 68. **Why are arteriovenous anastomoses (shunts) important in phasic activity of organs?**
Answer: Arteriovenous anastomoses (shunts) are important in phasic activity of organs because of following reason:
- They regulate blood flow.
- When an organ is active, these shunts are closed, and blood circulates through the capillaries.
- At rest, blood bypasses the capillary bed and is shunted back through the arteriovenous anastomosis.

Q. 69. Why do arteriovenous shunts possess a thick muscular coat and are under the influence of the sympathetic system?

Answer: Arteriovenous shunts possess a thick muscular coat and are under the influence of the sympathetic system because of following reason:
- To regulate their opening and closing, which controls blood flow through the shunt depending on the activity level of the organ.

Q. 70. Why are specialized arteriovenous anastomoses found in the skin of digital pads and nail beds?

Answer: Specialized arteriovenous anastomoses are found in the skin of digital pads and nail beds because of following reason:
- To regulate temperature by controlling blood flow, helping to conserve heat in cooler environments and dissipate heat in warmer conditions.

Q. 71. Why are preferential 'thoroughfare channels' considered a kind of shunt in the circulatory system?

Answer: Preferential 'thoroughfare channels' are considered a kind of shunt in the circulatory system because of following reason:
- They bypass the capillary network, with many true capillaries.
- They arise as side branches, forming microcirculatory units.
- They vary in size and activity depending on metabolic needs.

Q. 72. Why are arteries that do not anastomose with their neighbours called end arteries?

Answer: Arteries that do not anastomose with their neighbour are called end arteries because of following reason:
- They do not have alternative pathways for blood flow.
- They lead to serious consequences if they become occluded.

Cardiovascular system - special circulations and conditions

Q. 73. Why portal circulation is considered part of systemic circulation?

Answer: Portal circulation is considered part of systemic circulation because
- It involves the transportation of blood through a specific sequence of capillary beds.
- In portal circulation, blood flows from one set of capillaries in the digestive organs (through the hepatic portal vein) to another set of capillaries in the liver before returning to the heart.

- Despite this unique route, it is still part of the systemic circulation as it is involved in delivering
    - Nutrients,
    - Hormones, and
    - Other substances to the liver and ultimately to the rest of the body.

Q. 74. Why is the vein draining the first capillary network in portal circulation called a portal vein?

Answer: The vein draining the first capillary network in portal circulation is called a portal vein because of following reason:
- It branches like an artery to form the second set of capillaries or sinusoids.

Q. 75. Why are examples of portal circulation given as hepatic, hypothalamo-hypophyseal, and renal?

Answer: Examples of portal circulation are given as hepatic, hypothalamo-hypophyseal, and renal because of following reason:
- These are specific examples where blood passes through **two capillary beds** before entering systemic circulation, each serving unique physiological functions.

Q. 76. Why do occlusions of end arteries, such as the central branches of cerebral arteries and vasa recta of mesenteric arteries, cause serious nutritional disturbances?

Answer: Occlusions of end arteries, such as the central branches of cerebral arteries and vasa recta of mesenteric arteries, cause serious nutritional disturbances because of following reason:
- They supply tissues that lack collateral circulation, resulting in tissue death.

Q. 77. Why is occlusion of the central artery of the retina particularly devastating?

Answer: Occlusion of the central artery of the retina is particularly devastating because of following reason:
- It results in blindness due to the lack of anastomoses with other retinal arteries, which cannot compensate for the loss of blood flow.

Miscellaneous questions

Q. 78. Why do arteriovenous anastomoses develop rapidly during the early years but diminish in number in old age?

Answer: Arteriovenous anastomoses develop rapidly during the early years because of because of following reason:
- They are important in regulation of
  - Temperature and
  - Blood flow in growing tissues.
- But diminish in number in old age due to factors such as
  - Thickening, or
  - Narrowing,
  - Atrophy.

They reduce the functionality.

Q. 79. Why the endothelium is considered a key component of the vessel wall?

Answer: The endothelium is considered a key component of the vessel wall because of following reason:
- It plays several major physiological roles. They are
  - It Influences the blood flow,
  - It regulates diffusion of substances,
  - It promotes haemostasis,
  - It participates in inflammation,
  - And responding to mechanical forces.

Q. 80. Why do vasa vasorum exist in larger vessels?

Answer: Vasa vasorum exist in larger vessels because of following reason:
- To provide a vascular supply within the adventitia,
- Ensuring the nourishment of the tissues of the vessel wall beyond the reach of simple diffusion from the lumen.

Q. 81. Why is the regulation of body water and solutes by the kidney dependent on ultrafiltration of plasma in the glomeruli?

Answer: The regulation of body water and solutes by the kidney depends on ultrafiltration of plasma in the glomeruli because of following reason:
- The renal vasculature has strong autoregulation.
- Afferent arterioles have fenestrated endothelium with high permeability.
- These arterioles have specialized basement membranes and are covered by podocytes.
- Ultrafiltration helps maintain glomerular capillary pressure.
- Differential constriction of arterioles also supports this process.
- This regulation is essential for controlling blood pressure and volume.

Q. 82. **Why is the myocardium referred to as the muscular component of the heart?**

Answer: The myocardium is referred to as the muscular component of the heart because of following reason:
- It constitutes the bulk of the heart's tissues.
- It consists predominantly of cardiac muscle cells, which are responsible for generating the force needed to pump blood throughout the body.

Q. 83. **Why is the myocardium supplied by the coronary vessels?**

Answer: The myocardium is supplied by the coronary vessels because of following reason:
- It requires a rich blood supply of
    - Oxygen and
    - Nutrition to function effectively.
- It is essential for continuous contraction and relaxation of the heart muscle.

Q. 84. **Why anastomoses are considered shunts in the cardiovascular system?**

Answer: Anastomoses are considered shunts in the cardiovascular system because of following reason:
- They provide alternative pathways for blood flow,
- Allowing for bypassing or redistribution of blood depending on the body's needs.

Q. 85. **Why can some arteries be palpated through the skin?**

Answer: Some arteries can be palpated through the skin because of following reason:
- They are located close to the body's surface and have relatively firm walls.
- They have relatively large, elastic walls that can be compressed by the pressure of the fingers.
- Palpable arteries include
    - The common carotid,
    - Facial,
    - Brachial,
    - Radial,
    - Abdominal aorta,
    - Femoral,
    - Posterior tibial, and
    - Dorsalis pedis arteries.

Q. 86. Why are the nerves supplying an artery called Nervi vascularis?

Answer: The nerves supplying an artery are called n by ervi vascularis because of following reason:
- They are responsible for regulating the diameter of the artery and controlling blood flow.
- These nerves are mostly non-myelinated sympathetic fibers that function as vasoconstrictors.

Q. 87. Why are some nerve fibers myelinated in the arteries?

Answer: Some nerve fibers in the arteries are myelinated because of following reason:
- They are believed to be sensory, providing feedback about the condition of the artery's outer and inner coats.

Q. 88. Why is vasodilator innervation restricted to specific sites in arteries?

Answer: Vasodilator innervation is restricted to specific sites in arteries because of following reason:
- Vasodilator innervation is restricted to specific sites in arteries because different tissues and organs have varying needs for blood flow regulation.
- Vasodilator nerves are concentrated in areas where precise control of blood vessel diameter is crucial for maintaining optimal blood flow and pressure.
- This targeted innervation allows for efficient and localized adjustment of blood flow to meet the specific metabolic demands of different regions.
- Skeletal muscle vessels are dilated by cholinergic sympathetic nerves.
- Exocrine gland vessels are dilated on parasympathetic stimulation.
- Cutaneous vessels are dilated locally, producing flare or redness after an injury, through axon reflexes mediated by afferent impulses in cutaneous nerves.

Q. 89. Why is the flare or redness produced after an injury in the skin?

Answer: The flare or redness produced after an injury in the skin because of following reason:
- Due to local vasodilation of cutaneous vessels. Blood vessels in the area dilate, allowing more blood to flow to the injured site. This increased blood flow brings immune cells to the area. This helps healing and also causes the redness that is visible.
- This vasodilation is caused by afferent impulses in cutaneous nerves. It passes antidromically (proceeding or conducting in a direction opposite to the usual one) through their collaterals to the blood vessels. This process known as axon reflex.

Q. 90. **Why are the skeletal muscle vessels dilated by cholinergic sympathetic nerves?**

Answer: Skeletal muscle vessels are dilated by cholinergic sympathetic nerves because of following reason:
- To increase blood flow to the muscles during physical activity. It ensures adequate oxygen and nutrient delivery.

Q. 91. **Why do the vasa vasorum form a dense capillary network in the tunica adventitia?**

Answer: The vasa vasorum form a dense capillary network in the tunica adventitia because of following reason:
- They supply
    - The adventitia and
    - The outer part of the tunica media with nutrients.

Q. 92. **Why the nutrient vessels are called vasa vasorum important for the arteries?**

Answer: The nutrient vessels are called vasa vasorum important for the arteries because of following reason:
- Their capillary network supplies the adventitia and the outer part of the tunica media with necessary nutrients.

Q. 93. **Why is the diffusion from the luminal blood necessary for the inner parts of the arterial wall?**

Answer: The diffusion from the luminal blood necessary for the inner parts of the arterial wall because of following reason:
- These parts are not supplied by the vasa vasorum and therefore rely on luminal blood for nourishment.

Q. 94. **Why do the skeletal muscle vessels dilate when stimulated by cholinergic sympathetic nerves?**

Answer: The skeletal muscle vessels dilate when stimulated by cholinergic sympathetic nerves because of following reason:
- These nerves provide vasodilator innervation,
- Hence increasing blood flow to the muscles.

Q. 95. **Why are non-myelinated sympathetic fibers predominantly found in the nerves supplying an artery?**

Answer: Non-myelinated sympathetic fibers predominantly found in the nerves supplying an artery because of following reason:
- These fibers are vasoconstrictor in function.
- They regulate
    - The arterial diameter and
    - Blood flow.

Q. 96. **Why do minute veins accompany arteries to drain blood from the outer part of the arterial wall?**

Answer: Minute veins accompany arteries to drain blood from the outer part of the arterial wall because of following reason:
- They maintain proper blood circulation.
- They prevent accumulation of blood in the arterial walls.

Q. 97. **Why does the presence of lymphatics in the adventitia indicate an important function?**

Answer: The presence of lymphatics in the adventitia indicate an important function because of following reason:
- They help in draining excess fluid.
- They maintain tissue fluid balance in the arterial wall.

Q. 98. **Why is vasodilation produced locally in cutaneous vessels after an injury?**

Answer: Vasodilation produced locally in cutaneous vessels after an injury because of following reason:
- The afferent impulses in the cutaneous nerves pass antidromically to the blood vessels.
- They cause the axon reflex and results in redness.

Q. 99. **Why do large veins have dead space around them?**

Answer: Large veins have dead space around them because of following reason:
- To allow for their dilatation during increased venous return.
- This dead space commonly contains regional lymph nodes.

Q. 100. **Why are nerves distributed to veins in the same manner as to arteries?**

Answer: Nerves are distributed to veins in the same manner as to arteries because of following reason:
- Veins also require neural regulation of their functions.

Q. 101. **Why do capillaries begin after a transition zone of 50-100 microns beyond the precapillary sphincters?**

Answer: Capillaries begin after a transition zone of 50-100 microns beyond the precapillary sphincters because of following reason:
- To ensure that the true capillaries, without any smooth muscle cells.
- Provide the required microcirculation for nutrient and gas exchange.

Q. 102. **Why are capillaries replaced by cavernous spaces in the sex organs, splenic pulp, and placenta?**

Answer: Capillaries are replaced by cavernous spaces in the sex organs, splenic pulp, and placenta because of following reason:
- To accommodate the unique functional requirements of these organs, such as increased blood flow during arousal in sex organs.
- Immune function in the spleen and placenta.

Q. 103. **Why are continuous capillaries found in the skin, connective tissue, muscles, lung, and brain?**

Answer: Continuous capillaries are found in the skin, connective tissue, muscles, lung, and brain because of following reason:
- They allow the passage of small molecules (up to 10 microns in size) across their walls.
- Maintaining a selective barrier while permitting exchange.

Q. 104. **Why may sinusoids connect arterioles with venules or venules with venules?**

Answer: Sinusoids may connect arterioles with venules or venules with venules because of following reason:
- In organs like the spleen, bone marrow, and liver to allow for specialized functions such as
  - Filtration,
  - Storage, and
  - Exchange of blood components.

Q. 105. **Why is arterial anastomosis between arteries or their branches classified as actual or potential?**

Answer: Arterial anastomosis between arteries or their branches is classified as actual or potential because of following reason:
- Actual anastomoses involve arteries meeting end-to-end, such as in
    - Palmar arches,
    - Plantar arch,
    - Circle of Willis,
    - Intestinal arcades, and
    - Labial branches of facial arteries.
- Potential anastomoses occur between terminal arterioles and can dilate gradually for collateral circulation.

Q. 106. **Why may potential arterial anastomoses fail to compensate for the loss of a main artery during sudden occlusion?**

Answer: Potential arterial anastomoses may fail to compensate for the loss of a main artery during sudden occlusion because of following reason:
- They can dilate only gradually, which limits their ability to provide sufficient collateral circulation.
- Examples include the coronary arteries and cortical branches of cerebral arteries.

Q. 107. **Why does the number of active microcirculatory units vary from time to time?**

Answer: The number of active microcirculatory units varies from time to time because of following reasons:
- To adapt to changing metabolic demands.
- To meet tissue oxygenation requirements.

Q. 108. **Why are the central artery of the retina and labyrinthine artery of the internal ear examples of absolute end arteries?**

Answer: The central artery of the retina and labyrinthine artery of the internal ear are examples of absolute end arteries because of following reason:
- They do not anastomose with other arteries.
- They make tissue vulnerable to death if occluded.

Q. 109.   Why do arteries of the spleen, kidney, lungs, and metaphyses of long bones fall under the category of end arteries?

Answer: Arteries of the spleen, kidney, lungs, and metaphyses of long bones fall under the category of end arteries because of following reason:
- They lack significant anastomoses with neighboring arteries.
- They make tissue susceptible to death if their blood supply is interrupted.

Q. 110.   Why is the maximum pressure during ventricular systole called systolic pressure?

Answer: The maximum pressure during ventricular systole is called systolic pressure because of following reason:
- It is generated by the force of contraction of the heart.

Q. 111.   Why is the minimum pressure during ventricular diastole called diastolic pressure?

Answer: The minimum pressure during ventricular diastole is called diastolic pressure because of following reason:
- It is mainly due to arteriolar tone (peripheral resistance).

Q. 112.   Why does the heart have to pump blood against diastolic pressure?

Answer: The heart has to pump blood against diastolic pressure because of following reason:
- Which is a direct load on the heart, ensuring continuous circulation of blood throughout the body.

Q. 113.   Why the difference between systolic and diastolic pressure is called 'pulse pressure'?

Answer: The difference between systolic and diastolic pressure is called 'pulse pressure' because of following reason:
- It represents the force generated by each heartbeat.
- It, reflects the stroke volume and elasticity of the arteries.

Q. 114.   Why does arterial hemorrhage cause spurting of blood?

Answer: Arterial hemorrhage causes spurting of blood because of following reason:
- Arteries have higher pressure compared to veins.
- It leads to a forceful ejection of blood when they are injured.

Q. 115. **Why does arteriosclerosis in old age lead to a rise in systolic pressure?**
Answer: Arteriosclerosis in old age leads to a rise in systolic pressure because of following reason:
- The stiffening of arteries reduces their ability to expand and contract.
- It increases the pressure exerted by the blood on arterial walls.

Q. 116. **Why is Buerger's disease (thromboangitis obliterans) very painful?**
Answer: Buerger's disease (thromboangitis obliterans) is very painful because of following reason:
- It involves inflammation of small peripheral arteries of the legs.
- It affects young smokers and causing significant discomfort.

Q. 117. **Why does Raynaud's phenomenon cause spasmodic pallor of the fingers?**
Answer: Raynaud's phenomenon causes spasmodic pallor of the fingers because of following reason:
- Small arteries and arterioles are constricted due to to cold.
- This reduces blood flow to the fingers.

Q. 118. **Why can acute phlebothrombosis lead to embolism?**
Answer: Acute phlebothrombosis can lead to embolism because of following reason:
- A thrombus formed in the veins of the lower limbs may dislodge and flow through the bloodstream. It has capability to block other arteries.

Q. 119. **Why do varicose veins occur when the vein wall is subjected to increased pressure over a long time?**
Answer: Varicose veins occur when the vein wall is subjected to increased pressure over a long time because of following reason:
- This leads to atrophy of
    - Muscle and
    - Elastic tissue.
- This causes the vein to stretch and bulge.

Q. 120. **Why is venous congestion of the feet relieved by elevating them above the trunk?**
Answer: Venous congestion of the feet is relieved by elevating them above the trunk because of following reason:
- This position helps in venous return.
- It reduces pressure in the veins and relieving tiredness.

Q. 121. **Why can parenteral nutrition be given through the right subclavian vein?**

Answer: Parenteral nutrition can be given through the right subclavian vein because of following reason:
- It provides direct access to the bloodstream.
- It allows the nutrients to quickly reach the circulatory system.

Q. 122. **Why is examination of blood vessels in the retina important in cases of diabetes and hypertension?**

Answer: Examination of blood vessels in the retina with an ophthalmoscope is important in cases of diabetes and hypertension because of following reason:
- To assess the health of the vessels.
- It helps to detect early signs of damage or disease.

Q. 123. **Why is the cardiovascular system essential for the body?**

Answer: The cardiovascular system is essential because of following reason:
- It supplies nutrients to and removes waste products from various tissues.
- It ensures the proper functioning of body.

Q. 124. **Why is blood considered the conveying medium in the cardiovascular system?**

Answer: Blood is considered the conveying medium because of following reason:
- It flows through blood vessels.
- It transports
    - Nutrients,
    - Oxygen,
    - Carbon dioxide, and
    - Other substances throughout the body.

Q. 125. **Why does the heart play a major role in the cardiovascular system?**

Answer: Heart play a major role in the cardiovascular system because of following reason:
- It pumps the blood.
- It provides the force necessary for blood circulation throughout the body.

Q. 126. **Why do arteries and veins have different functions in the cardiovascular system?**

Answer: Arteries and veins have different functions because of following reason:
- Arteries carry blood away from the heart to the tissues.
- Veins return blood from the tissues back to the heart.

Q. 127. **Why are capillaries important in the cardiovascular system?**

Answer: Capillaries are important in the cardiovascular system because of following reason:
- They connect arteries and veins.
- They allow the exchange of
    - Nutrients,
    - Metabolites, and
    - Respiratory gases like
        - Oxygen and
        - Carbon dioxide between blood and tissues.

Q. 128. **Why do lymphocytes mature in different locations, such as bone marrow and thymus?**

Answer: Lymphocytes mature in different locations, such as bone marrow and thymus, because of following reason:
- Each type of lymphocyte, B cells and T cells, requires specific environments.
- They signal to become
    - Immunocompetent and
    - Fully functional in the immune response.

Q. 129. **Why do arteries not have valves in their lumen?**

Answer: Arteries do not have valves in their lumen because of following reason:
- The pressure in the arteries is high.
- The blood directly pumped from the heart.
- It is sufficient to ensure unidirectional blood flow.

Q. 130. **Why is the regulation of regional blood flow a function of arteriovenous anastomoses?**

Answer: The regulation of regional blood flow is a function of arteriovenous anastomoses because of following reason:
- They bypass capillary beds.
- They allow the adjustment of blood distribution to specific areas as needed.

Q. 131. **Why do the erectile tissues of sex organs have arteriovenous anastomoses?**

Answer: The erectile tissues of sex organs have arteriovenous anastomoses because of following reason:
- To facilitate rapid blood flow.
- It is required for sexual arousal and function.

Q. 132.   Why are the thick muscular walls of arteriovenous shunts essential?

Answer: The thick muscular walls of arteriovenous shunts are essential because of following reason:
- They provide the structural strength needed to regulate blood flow and pressure through contraction and relaxation.

Q. 133.   Why do the collapsed fetal lungs necessitate a different circulatory pattern compared to adults?

Answer: The collapsed fetal lungs necessitate a different circulatory pattern compared to adults because of following reason:
- They are not yet functional for gas exchange.
- They require blood to be oxygenated through the placenta.

Q. 134.   Why does the left heart pump blood through both systemic circulation and the placenta in fetal circulation?

Answer: The left heart pump blood through both systemic circulation and the placenta in fetal circulation because of following reason:
- The left heart pumps blood through both systemic circulation and the placenta in fetal circulation.
- This is to ensure that oxygenated blood reaches the entire body and returns to the placenta for re-oxygenation.

Q. 135.   Why do the shunts in fetal circulation close down postnatally?

Answer: The shunts in fetal circulation close down postnatally because of following reason:
- The lungs and liver become fully functional after birth.
- This allow the circulatory system to transit to the adult pattern of blood flow.

Q. 136.   Why is Hering's Nerve significant in cardiovascular physiology?

Answer: Hering's Nerve, the carotid sinus branch of the glossopharyngeal nerve, is significant because of following reason:
- It forms the afferent limb of the carotid sinus reflex.
- It helps regulate blood pressure by sensing changes in arterial wall stretch.

6. Nervous system

Central nervous system (CNS)

Q. 1. Why does the central nervous system (CNS) include the brain and spinal cord?

Answer: The central nervous system includes the brain and spinal cord because of following reason:
- These structures
    - Integrate and process sensory information,
    - Initiate and coordinate motor responses, and are
    - Essential for higher cognitive functions.

Q. 2. Why are the bundles of nerve fibers within the central nervous system called tracts?

Answer: The bundles of nerve fibers within the central nervous system are called tracts because of following reason:
- They are collections of axons that have a similar origin, destination, and function.

Q. 3. Why are the fibers of the CNS myelinated by oligodendrocytes, while those of the PNS are myelinated by Schwann cells?

Answer: The fibers of the central nervous system (CNS) are myelinated by oligodendrocytes, while those of the peripheral nervous system (PNS) are myelinated by Schwann cells because of following reason:
- The different embryological origins and structures of these two types of glial cells.
- The fibers of the CNS are myelinated by oligodendrocytes.
- Myelination of peripheral nervous system is done by Schwann cells.
- The glial cells are specialized for different parts of the nervous system.
- Oligodendrocytes in the CNS can myelinate multiple nerve fibers at once.
- They make them efficient for the dense network of neurons in the brain and spinal cord.
- Schwann cells in the PNS, on the other hand, myelinate only one nerve fiber per cell.
- It provides insulation and support for the peripheral nerves that connect the CNS to the rest of the body.
- The division of labor ensures that both the central and peripheral nervous systems function effectively.

Q. 4.   **Why do oligodendrocytes in the CNS form myelin sheaths around several axons?**

Answer: Oligodendrocytes in the CNS form myelin sheaths around several axons because of following reason:
- They can extend their processes to wrap multiple axons simultaneously.
- This allows them to efficiently provide myelin insulation for the densely packed neurons in the CNS.
- By myelinating several axons, oligodendrocytes optimize space and resources, ensuring rapid signal transmission across the complex neural network of the brain and spinal cord.
- This arrangement supports the high density and connectivity of neural pathways in the central nervous system.

Q. 5.   **Why do certain dyes fail to stain the parenchyma of the brain and spinal cord when injected intravenously?**

Answer: Certain dyes fail to stain the parenchyma of the brain and spinal cord when injected intravenously because of following reason:
- They are unable to pass through the blood-brain barrier at the capillary level.

Q. 6.   **Why do the same dyes, when injected into the ventricles, enter the brain substances easily?**

Answer: The same dyes, when injected into the ventricles, enter the brain substances easily because of following reason:
- The ventricular system is not protected by the blood-brain barrier, allowing substances to directly access the brain tissue.

Q. 7.   **Why does the presence of the blood-brain barrier indicate a barrier at the capillary level between the blood and nerve cells?**

Answer: The presence of the blood-brain barrier indicates a barrier at the capillary level between the blood and nerve cells because of following reason:
- It is a specialized system of endothelial cells that tightly regulate the exchange of substances between the bloodstream and the brain.
- This barrier consists of tightly joined endothelial cells in the capillaries of the brain.
- It prevents
    - Large molecules,
    - Toxins, and
    - Pathogens from entering the brain.
    - It allows necessary nutrients to pass through.

o This selective permeability protects the brain from harmful substances and maintains a stable environment for neural function

Q. 8. Why is the blood-brain barrier important in the nervous system?
Answer: The blood-brain barrier is important in the nervous system because of following reason:
- It protects the brain from potentially harmful substances, such as toxins and pathogens, while allowing essential nutrients to pass through.
- It maintains a stable environment for proper neuronal function by regulating the movement of ions and molecules.
- This selective permeability helps preserve the brain's delicate balance and supports its overall health and function.

Q. 9. Why are capillary endothelium without fenestrations, basement membrane, and the end feet of astrocytes considered components of the blood-brain barrier?
Answer: Capillary endothelium without fenestrations, a basement membrane, and the end feet of astrocytes are considered components of the blood-brain barrier because of following reason:
- They work together to restrict the movement of substances between the blood and the brain.
- **Capillary endothelium without fenestrations**: the endothelial cells in brain capillaries have tightly joined junctions. It prevents large molecules and potentially harmful substances from passing through.
- **Basement membrane**: this provides structural support and further limits permeability, contributing to the barrier's selective nature.
- **End feet of astrocytes**: these glial cells wrap around the capillaries. They help to regulate the barrier's permeability by releasing factors that influence the tight junctions between endothelial cells.
- Together, these components create a protective barrier that maintains the brain's stable environment.

Q. 10. Why is each spinal nerve connected to the spinal cord by two roots?
Answer: Each spinal nerve is connected to the spinal cord by two roots because of following reason:
- A ventral root, which is motor, and a dorsal root, which is sensory, because this arrangement allows for the integration of motor and sensory functions within the nerve.

Q. 11.   **Why is the dorsal root characterized by the presence of a spinal ganglion?**
Answer: The dorsal root is characterized by the presence of a spinal ganglion because of following reason:
- Contains cell bodies of sensory neurons that convey sensory information from the periphery to the central nervous system.

Q. 12.   **Why is the vertebral foramen important?**
Answer: Vertebral foramen important because of following reason:
- It contains
    - The spinal cord,
    - Cauda equina,
    - Spinal meninges,
    - Spinal arteries, and
    - The internal vertebral venous plexus, the vertebral foramen indicates its crucial role in protecting and supporting the central nervous system and its associated structures.

Peripheral nervous system (PNS)

Q. 13.   **Why peripheral nerves and ganglia are considered part of the peripheral nervous system (PNS)?**
Answer: Peripheral nerves and ganglia are considered part of the peripheral nervous system because of following reason:
- They are located outside the central nervous system.
- They transmit sensory information to the CNS.
- They send motor commands from the CNS to muscles and glands.

Q. 14.   **Why the axons of nerve cells are called nerve fibers?**
Answer: The axons of nerve cells are called nerve fibers because of following reason:

- They are long, slender projections.
- They conduct electrical impulses away from the cell body of neuron.

Q. 15.   **Why are the bundles of nerve fibers in the peripheral nervous system called peripheral nerves or simply nerves?**
Answer: The bundles of nerve fibers in the peripheral nervous system are called peripheral nerves or simply nerves because of following reason:
- They contain axons bundled together with connective tissue.
- They serve to transmit signals between the central nervous system and the rest of the body.

Q. 16.   Why are nonmyelinated fibers surrounded by Schwann cells in the PNS?

Answer: Nonmyelinated fibers are surrounded by Schwann cells in the peripheral nervous system (PNS) because of following reason:
- Schwann cells form indentations that envelop several axons, providing support and some insulation to these axons.

Q. 17.   Why nerves are considered solid white cords?

Answer: Nerves are considered solid white cords because of following reason:
- They are composed of bundles (fasciculi) of nerve fibers, which are surrounded by connective tissue sheaths. These sheaths give nerves their solid appearance.

Q. 18.   Why is each nerve fiber delicate and friable despite the toughness of the nerve?

Answer: Each nerve fiber is delicate and friable despite the toughness of the nerve because of following reason:
- Nerve fibers are composed mainly of axons, which are delicate structures responsible for transmitting nerve impulses.
- The toughness of the nerve comes from the fibrous sheaths (epineurium, perineurium, and endoneurium) that surround and protect the nerve fibers.

Q. 19.   Why is the whole nerve trunk ensheathed by epineurium?

Answer: The whole nerve trunk is ensheathed by epineurium because of following reason:
- To provide protection and structural support to the nerve as a whole. It forms the outermost layer of connective tissue around the nerve.

Q. 20.   Why is each fasciculus ensheathed by perineurium?

Answer: Each fasciculus is ensheathed by perineurium because of following reason:
- To protect and support the bundles of nerve fibers within the nerve.
- Perineurium is a connective tissue sheath that surrounds each fascicle.

Q. 21.   Why is each nerve fiber ensheathed by endoneurium?

Answer: Each nerve fiber is ensheathed by endoneurium because of following reason:
- To provide a delicate and supportive covering. Endoneurium is a delicate connective tissue layer that surrounds individual nerve fibers within a fascicle.

Q. 22.   Why do the ventral and dorsal nerve roots unite within the intervertebral foramen to form the spinal nerve?

Answer: The ventral and dorsal nerve roots unite within the intervertebral foramen to form the spinal nerve because of following reason:

- This union integrates both motor and sensory functions, facilitating communication between the central nervous system and the periphery.

Q. 23. Why does the dorsal ramus of the spinal nerve supply the intrinsic muscles of the back and the skin covering them?

Answer: The dorsal ramus of the spinal nerve supplies the intrinsic muscles of the back and the skin covering them because of following reason:
- It branches off posteriorly to innervate the structures located dorsally along the spinal column.

Q. 24. Why are the ventral rami of some spinal nerves plaited to form nerve plexuses for the limbs?

Answer: The ventral rami of some spinal nerves are plaited to form nerve plexuses for the limbs because of following reason:
- This arrangement allows for the mixing and redistribution of nerve fibers, facilitating the complex innervation patterns required for limb movement and sensation.

Q. 25. Why are nerve plexuses formed only by the ventral rami and never by the dorsal rami?

Answer: Nerve plexuses are formed only by the ventral rami and never by the dorsal rami because of following reason:
- The ventral rami contain the majority of the motor and sensory fibers that innervate the limbs, facilitating coordinated movement and sensation.

Autonomic nervous system (ANS)

Q. 26. Why does the autonomic nervous system include both sympathetic and parasympathetic nervous systems?

Answer: The autonomic nervous system includes both the sympathetic and parasympathetic nervous systems because of following reason:
- They work together to maintain balance in the body's involuntary functions.
- The sympathetic system prepares the body for "fight or flight" responses,
- The parasympathetic system promotes "rest and digest" activities.
- This dual system allows the body to respond to different situations effectively and maintain homeostasis.

Q. 27. **Why are myelinated fibers examples of nerve fibers in the somatic nervous system more than 1 μm in diameter and all preganglionic fibers of the autonomic nervous system?**

Answer: Myelinated fibers are examples of nerve fibers in the somatic nervous system more than 1 μm in diameter and all preganglionic fibers of the autonomic nervous system because of following reason:
- These fibers require fast conduction of nerve impulses for rapid and efficient transmission of sensory and motor signals.

Q. 28. **Why are unmyelinated nerve fibers examples of nerve fibers in the somatic nervous system less than 1 μm in diameter and all postganglionic fibers of the autonomic nervous system?**

Answer: Unmyelinated nerve fibers are examples of nerve fibers in the somatic nervous system less than 1 μm in diameter and all postganglionic fibers of the autonomic nervous system because of following reason:
- They do not require rapid conduction of nerve impulses and are involved in more diffuse, slower transmission of signals.

Q. 29. **Why is Langley's Ganglion important in autonomic nervous system studies?**

Answer: Langley's Ganglion, or the submandibular ganglion, is important because of following reason:
- It relays parasympathetic innervation to the submandibular and sublingual glands, indicating its role in saliva production and autonomic regulation.

Q. 30. **Why is sympathectomy sometimes helpful in relieving symptoms of vasospasmodic diseases of the limbs?**

Answer: Sympathectomy is beneficial in conditions like Buerger's disease and Raynaud's disease because of following reason:
- The sympathetic system, responsible for blood vessel constriction, is inhibited. Hence, dilating the blood vessels improves circulation and alleviates symptoms of ischemia.

Neurons and neuroglia

Q. 31. **Why does neuroglia provide structural and functional support to neurons?**

Answer: Neuroglia provide structural and functional support to neurons because of following reason:
- They maintain the microenvironment around neurons.
- They support their metabolic needs.
- They participate in the repair process after injury.

Q. 32. **Why neurons are considered the structural and functional units of the nervous system?**

Answer: Neurons are considered the structural and functional units of the nervous system because of following reason:
- The structure and function of a dendrite, cell body, and axon of neuron are consistent across all neurons in the body. Because of this consistency a neuron is regarded as the structural and functional unit of the nervous system.
- Neurons are the basic cells.
- They make up the nervous system.
- They are responsible for transmitting signals throughout the body.
- They carry out the essential functions of receiving, processing, and sending information, which allows the nervous system to control and coordinate bodily activities

Q. 33. **Why do neurons exhibit excitability and conductivity?**

Answer: Neurons exhibit excitability and conductivity because of following reason:
- They need to respond to stimuli and transmit electrical signals efficiently.
- Excitability allows neurons to generate an action potential in response to a stimulus.
- Conductivity enables them to carry this electrical signal along their length to communicate with other neurons, muscles, or glands.
- These properties are essential for neurons to perform their role in transmitting information within the nervous system.

Q. 34. **Why are dendrites important in a neuron's function?**

Answer: Dendrites are important in a neuron's function because of following reason:
- They receive impulses from other neurons and transmit them toward the cell body for integration.

Q. 35. **Why does the axon of a neuron not branch except at its termination?**

Answer: The axon of a neuron does not branch except at its termination because of following reason:
- Its primary function is to transmit a signal from the cell body to a specific target, such as another neuron or muscle cell.
- By branching only at the termination, the axon ensures that the signal is directed to the correct location without interference, allowing for precise communication within the nervous system.

Q. 36. **Why are pseudo unipolar neurons classified as sensory neurons?**
Answer: Pseudo unipolar neurons are classified as sensory neurons because of following reason:
- Their single process divides into
    - A central branch (axon) that carries impulses to the central nervous system and
    - A peripheral branch (dendrite) that receives sensory information.

Q. 37. **Why are multipolar neurons the most common type in the nervous system?**
Answer: Multipolar neurons are the most common type in the nervous system because of following reason:
- They have several dendrites and one axon, which allows them to integrate and transmit information to multiple target cells.

Q. 38. **Why do Golgi type I neurons have long axons?**
Answer: Golgi type I neurons have long axons, up to 1 meter long, because of following reason:
- They transmit nerve impulses over long distances, such as from
    - The brain to the spinal cord or
    - From the spinal cord to peripheral muscles.

Q. 39. **Why pyramidal cells are shaped the way they are?**
Answer: Pyramidal cells are shaped with a cone/pyramidal-shaped cell body because of following reason:
- Their dendrites arise from the angles of the cone, allowing them to integrate information in a specific direction.

Q. 40. **Why do stellate cells have dendrites extending in all directions from the cell body?**
Answer: Stellate cells have dendrites extending in all directions from the cell body because of following reason:
- They receive input from multiple sources.
- They integrate information locally within the cerebellar cortex and sympathetic ganglia.

Q. 41. **Why are amacrine cells important in the retina of the eye?**

Answer: Amacrine cells are important in the retina of the eye because of following reason:
- They play a crucial role in processing visual information. They modulate and integrate signals between bipolar cells and ganglion cells, which helps refine the visual input before it is transmitted to the brain. This contributes to important visual functions like detecting motion, adjusting to changes in light, and enhancing image contrast.

Q. 42. **Why do Schwann cells myelinate only 1 mm of axon, leaving gaps in the myelin sheath called nodes of Ranvier?**

Answer: Schwann cells myelinate only 1 mm of axon, leaving gaps in the myelin sheath called nodes of Ranvier, because of following reason:
- These gaps allow for saltatory conduction.
- The nerve impulse jumps from node to node, speeding up the conduction of the nerve impulse.

Q. 43. **Why is dynamic polarity observed in neurons?**

Answer: Dynamic polarity is observed in neurons because of following reason:
- Impulses flow towards the cell body in the dendrites and away from the cell body in the axon, allowing for efficient transmission of signals.

Q. 44. **Why are synapses important in the nervous system?**

Answer: Synapses are important in the nervous system because of following reason:
- They are junctions between neurons where information is transmitted from one neuron to another via neurotransmitters.
- It enables communication and processing of signals.

Q. 45. **Why glial cells are considered non-excitable cells in the nervous system?**

Answer: Glial cells are considered non-excitable cells in the nervous system because of following reason:
- They do not generate or conduct electrical impulses.
- They are essential for support of neurons.

Q. 46. **Why are astrocytes, oligodendrocytes, and microglia important in the nervous system?**

Answer: Astrocytes, oligodendrocytes, and microglia are important in the nervous system because of following reason:
- They provide
    - Mechanical support to neurons,
    - Insulate them,
    - Remove debris,
    - Maintain the ionic environment, and
    - Myelinate nerve fibers, contributing to neuronal health and function.

Q. 47. **Why do myelinated nerves have a sheath of myelin between the axis cylinder and neurilemma?**

Answer: Myelinated nerves have a sheath of myelin between the axis cylinder and neurilemma because of following reason:
- To insulate the nerve fiber and increase the speed of electrical signal transmission.
- Myelin, produced by Schwann cells in the Pns and oligodendrocytes in the CNS, acts as an insulating layer that prevents electrical impulses from leaking out of the axon and allows them to travel more quickly along the nerve fiber.
- The neurilemma, the outermost layer of the Schwann cell in the Pns, provides additional support and protection to the myelin sheath and axon.

Q. 48. **Why are non-myelinated nerve fibers important in the nervous system?**

Answer: Non-myelinated nerve fibers important in the nervous system because of following reason:
- Remak's fibers conduct impulses more slowly and are found in autonomic nerves, they indicate their role in regulating involuntary functions such as digestion and heart rate.

* Remak's fiber" is a glial-neurite complex, i.e. A bundle of unmyelinated nerve fibers covered with a single glial cell.

Q. 49. **Why are microglia considered the smallest neuroglia?**

Answer: Microglia considered the smallest neuroglia because of following reason:
- They are small, mobile cells that act as the primary immune defence in the central nervous system.

Reflexes and Functional Units

Q. 50. **Why a reflex arc is considered the basic functional unit of the nervous system?**

Answer: A reflex arc is considered the basic functional unit of the nervous system because of following reason:
- It can perform integrated neural activity independently of conscious thought or control.

Q. 51. **Why a monosynaptic reflex arc is simpler compared to a polysynaptic reflex arc?**

Answer: A monosynaptic reflex arc is simpler compared to a polysynaptic reflex arc because of following reason:
- It involves only two neurons: a sensory (afferent) neuron and a motor (efferent) neuron, connected by a single synapse.
- In contrast, a polysynaptic reflex arc includes one or more interneurons (internuncial neurons) between the sensory and motor neurons, which adds complexity to the pathway.

Q. 52. **Why does a monosynaptic reflex arc involve only a sensory neuron and a motor neuron?**

Answer: A monosynaptic reflex arc involves only a sensory neuron and a motor neuron because of following reason:
- The reflex response is rapid and simple, requiring minimal processing. This allows for quick responses to stimuli, such as in stretch reflexes (tendon jerks).

Q. 53. **Why the withdrawal reflex is considered a polysynaptic reflex?**

Answer: The withdrawal reflex (response to a painful stimulus) is considered a polysynaptic reflex because of following reason:
- It involves additional interneurons (internuncial neurons) between the sensory neuron carrying the pain signal and the motor neurons causing the withdrawal of the limb from the painful stimulus.

Q. 54. **Why stretch are reflexes (tendon jerks) examples of monosynaptic reflexes?**

Answer: Stretch reflexes (tendon jerks) are examples of monosynaptic reflexes because of following reason:
- They involve a direct connection between the sensory neuron (afferent neuron) from the muscle spindle and the motor neuron (efferent neuron) to the muscle. There is no involvement of interneurons.

Segmental innervation and nerve plexuses

Q. 55. **Why do limb plexuses come from the anterior primary rami of spinal nerves?**

Answer: The anterior primary rami supply the skin at the sides and front of the neck and body because of following reason:
- They branch from the spinal nerves that emerge from the spinal cord.
- These rami carry sensory and motor fibers to the front and sides of the body, including the skin. Their distribution pattern allows them to innervate the skin in these regions, providing sensation and contributing to motor control.

Q. 56. **Why are dermatomes important in understanding segmental supply of skin and sympathetic nerve distribution?**

Answer: Dermatomes are clinically important because of following reason:
- They map the segmental supply of the skin by spinal nerves.
- They help identify the specific spinal nerve or spinal cord segment responsible for sensory innervation in different skin areas.
- Understanding dermatomes also aids in diagnosing nerve or spinal cord injuries.
- It also help to understand the distribution of sympathetic nerves to the skin.

Q. 57. **Why is segmental innervation of muscles considered to be based on 4 underlying facts?**

Answer: Segmental innervation of muscles is considered to be based on four underlying facts because of following reason:
1. **Embryological development:** Muscles develop from somites, which are segmented blocks of mesoderm along the spinal cord. Each somite is associated with a specific spinal nerve, establishing a segmental pattern.
2. **Nerve growth:** Spinal nerves grow out to innervate the muscles derived from their corresponding somite. It preserves the segmental organization.
3. **Functional grouping:** Muscles are often grouped based on their segmental innervation, with each group receiving input from a specific spinal segment or a few adjacent segments.
4. **Clinical correlation:** The segmental pattern helps in clinical diagnosis, as muscle weakness or paralysis in a specific group can indicate damage to the corresponding spinal nerve or segment.

Q. 58. **Why are most muscles supplied equally from two adjacent segments?**

Answer: Most muscles are supplied equally from two adjacent segments because of following reason:
- To ensure efficient motor control and redundancy in innervation.
- This arrangement allows for continuous function even if one segment is damaged.
- It provides backup support and smooth muscle coordination.

Q. 59. **Why do muscles sharing a common primary action on a joint receive innervation from the same segments?**

Answer: Muscles sharing a common primary action on a joint receive innervation from the same segments because of following reason:
- To coordinate their movements efficiently.
- This arrangement ensures that muscles working together for a specific action are controlled simultaneously.
- It allows for smooth and synchronized joint movement.
- It also simplifies the nervous system's control over related muscle groups.

Q. 60. **Why do spinal centers for joint movements tend to occupy four continuous segments in the cord?**

Answer: Spinal centers for joint movements tend to occupy four continuous segments in the spinal cord because of following reason:
- To provide a broader range of control and coordination for complex movements.
- This distribution ensures that multiple muscles involved in a joint's movement are innervated across several segments. It allows for more precise and synchronized motor control.
- It also offers redundancy, so if one segment is damaged, others can still contribute to the movement.

Q. 61. **Why does the segmental innervation lie lower in the spinal cord for joints more distal in the limb?**

Answer: The segmental innervation lies lower in the spinal cord for joints more distal in the limb because of the way the spinal cord segments map to the body.
- As one moves from proximal to distal regions of the limb, the spinal cord segments controlling these areas are positioned lower.
- This reflects the developmental pattern where the spinal nerves that innervate distal parts of the limbs originate from lower segments of the spinal cord.

Q. 62. **Why the movements of the lower limb are summarized based on pairs of recited numbers?**

Answer: The movements of the lower limb are summarized based on pairs of recited numbers because of following reason:
- To simplify the understanding and description of complex joint actions. This method groups movements into pairs that work together, making it easier to remember and analyse their interactions.

Q. 63. **Why inversion and eversion of the foot are considered movements innervated by a single segment?**

Answer: Inversion and eversion of the foot are considered movements innervated by a single segment because of following reason:
- To demonstrate the specificity of innervation patterns in the lower limb.

Q. 64. Why does the upper limb conform to the general plan of segmental innervation?

Answer: Inversion and eversion of the foot are considered movements innervated by a single segment because of following reason:
- They are primarily controlled by the muscles that receive their nerve supply from a specific segment of the spinal cord.
- Inversion, which involves turning the sole of the foot inward.
- Eversion, which involves turning it outward.
- They are mainly controlled by the tibial nerve (for inversion) and the peroneal nerve (for eversion), which originate from the same spinal nerve segments (l4-l5 and s1-s2).
- Thus, these movements are linked to the function of a single segment of the spinal cord.

Q. 65. Why do movements below the elbow not always conform to the pattern of four spinal segments for each joint?

Answer: Movements below the elbow do not always conform to the pattern of four spinal segments for each joint because of following reason:
- The innervation of muscles in the forearm and hand comes from multiple nerve roots and peripheral nerves, rather than a strict segmental pattern.
- Muscles involved in these movements are innervated by nerves that originate from different spinal segments and can overlap in their contributions.
- Additionally, some muscles are innervated by nerves that span more than one spinal segment, leading to a more complex and integrated control system rather than a simple four-segment pattern for each joint.

Miscellaneous questions

Q. 66. Why are there 2 types of nerve fibers found in the nervous system, myelinated and nonmyelinated?

Answer: There are two types of nerve fibers, myelinated and nonmyelinated, in the nervous system because of following reason:
- Each type serves different functions in transmitting nerve signals.
- Myelinated fibers are covered with a fatty layer called myelin.
- They increase the speed of conduction of electrical impulses.
- This is crucial for rapid responses, such as reflexes and quick motor movements.
- Nonmyelinated fibers lack this coating and transmit signals more slowly, which is suitable for functions that do not require immediate response, like regulating internal organs.
- Therefore, the nervous system uses both types to efficiently handle different physiological processes.

Q. 67. **Why does myelination of a peripheral nerve fiber occur in the way described?**

Answer: Myelination of a peripheral nerve fiber occurs in the way described because of following reason:
- Schwann cells wrap around a single nerve fiber, creating a thick, protective myelin sheath.
- This process involves Schwann cells extending their membrane around the nerve fiber multiple times.
- This tight wrapping increases the speed of electrical impulse transmission along the fiber, essential for efficient communication between the CNS and peripheral tissues.
- The single-cell myelination strategy ensures that each peripheral nerve fiber receives individual support and insulation, crucial for the proper functioning of the peripheral nervous system.

Q. 68. **Why is the nervous system described as having a simple plan?**

Answer: The nervous system is described as having a simple plan because of following reason:
- Its basic structure and function are fundamentally straightforward.
- It consists of neurons, which transmit electrical signals, and glial cells, which support and protect neurons.
- The core functional units are
    - Sensory input,
    - Integration, and
    - Motor output.
- This simplicity in organization allows the nervous system to perform complex tasks through basic, repetitive processes.
- Despite its complexity in terms of connectivity and function, its fundamental structure remains relatively simple.

Q. 69. **Why are nerve cells described as conducting impulses in only one direction?**

Answer: Nerve cells are described as conducting impulses in only one direction because of following reason:
- The processes conveying impulses to the nerve cell are called dendrites, while the process conveying the impulse away from the nerve cell is called an axon.

Q. 70. **Why cell bodies with similar functions are tend to group themselves together into ganglia or nuclei?**

Answer: Cell bodies with similar functions tend to group themselves together into ganglia or nuclei because of following reason:
- To optimize processing and coordination.

- In these clusters, neurons can
    - Efficiently communicate with each other,
    - Integrate information, and
    - Produce coordinated responses.
- This organization simplifies the management of complex processes by localizing related functions and streamlining neural circuits, enhancing the efficiency and effectiveness of neural processing.

Q. 71. Why are nerves in the limbs supplied by branches from local arteries?

Answer: Nerves in the limbs are supplied by branches from local arteries because of following reason:
- These arteries provide the necessary oxygen and nutrients to the nerves. They maintain proper function of these arteries.
- The close relations of these arteries to the nerves allows for
    - Efficient and
    - Localized blood supply,
- It is crucial for
    - Maintaining nerve health and
    - Facilitating nerve signal transmission.

Q. 72. Why does the nerve supply to a part not alter after it is established in the embryo?

Answer: The nerve supply to a part not alter after it is established in the embryo because of following reason:
- The nerve supply to a part does not alter after it is established in the embryo to maintain consistent neurological function throughout life.

Q. 73. Why do the anterior primary rami supply the skin at the sides and front of the neck and body?

Answer: The anterior primary rami supply the skin at the sides and front of the neck and body because of following reason:
- During embryological development, the ventral (anterior) portion of the embryo gives rise to these structures.
- As the embryo develops, the spinal nerves differentiate into dorsal and ventral (anterior) rami.
- The anterior primary rami extend to innervate the muscles and skin of the front and sides of the body. It follows the pattern established during early development.
- This embryological origin determines the areas they supply in the adult body.

Q. 74. **Why flexor muscles of the upper limb are supplied by nerve branches from the extensor compartment?**

Answer: Flexor muscles of the upper limb are supplied by nerve branches from the extensor compartment because of following reason:
- Flexor muscles are sometimes supplied by branches of nerve of the extensor compartment.
- This is as per nerve development during embryological growth. Nerves grow toward their target muscles as they develop.
- These pathways can cross compartments.
- As a result, some nerve branches may originate from the extensor compartment but continue to supply flexor muscles.
- This arrangement is a result of the complex migration and growth patterns of muscles and nerves during embryogenesis.

Q. 75. **Why is the flexor compartment of the limb supplied by a richer nerve supply compared to the extensor compartment?**

Answer: The flexor compartment of the limb is supplied by a richer nerve supply compared because of following reason:
- To the extensor compartment because flexor muscles are more precise in movement and require finer control, which is facilitated by a richer nerve supply.

Q. 76. **Why plexus formation is considered a physiological or functional adaptation?**

Answer: Plexus formation is considered a physiological or functional adaptation because of following reason:
- It allows for the precise and coordinated innervation necessary for complex limb movements, integrating various nerve fibers to support limb function effectively.

Q. 77. **Why are telephone numbers usually seven digits long?**

Answer: Telephone numbers are typically seven digits long because of following reason:
- Short-term memory, which retains information for a few seconds to minutes, can generally hold about seven bits of information.
- Therefore, grouping numbers into segments separated by spaces, such as area codes, allows for easier recall within this memory capacity.

7. Skin and fascia

Epidermal layer (keratinocytes, melanocytes, merkel cells)

Q. 1. **Why do melanocytes produce melanin pigment?**
Answer: Melanocytes produce melanin pigment because of following reason:
- To protect the skin from the harmful effects of ultraviolet (UV) radiation.
- Melanin absorbs and disperses UV rays, reducing the risk of DNA damage in skin cells.
- It helps to prevent skin cancer.
- It also gives color to the skin, hair, and eyes.

Q. 2. **Why do ectodermal cells differentiate mainly into keratinocytes and probably Merkel cells?**
Answer: Ectodermal cells differentiate mainly into keratinocytes and Merkel cells because of following reason:
- These cell types are essential for the skin's functions.
- Keratinocytes form the primary protective layer of the epidermis. It produces keratin that
    - Strengthens and
    - Protects the skin.
- Merkel cells, although less abundant. They are involved in sensory functions, specifically touch and pressure sensation.
- This differentiation is crucial for the skin's role in protection, sensation, and maintaining homeostasis.

Q. 3. **Why do nerves and associated Schwann cells enter and traverse the dermis during development?**
Answer: Nerves and associated Schwann cells enter and traverse the dermis during development because of following reason:
- To establish the sensory and autonomic nerve networks necessary for skin function.
- Schwann cells provide support and insulation to nerve fibers, facilitating efficient signal transmission.
- This network allows the skin to detect and respond to various stimuli, such as touch, temperature, and pain, and plays a role in regulating blood flow and other skin functions.

Q. 4. **Why does the epidermis develop into a bilaminar epithelium during embryonic development?**

Answer: The epidermis develops into a bilaminar epithelium during embryonic development to because of following reason:
- Establish 2 distinct layers:
  - The periderm and
  - The basal layer.
- The periderm acts as a temporary protective layer, while the basal layer forms the foundation for the future stratified epidermis.
- This bilaminar structure is crucial for initial skin formation and protection as the fetus develops, eventually giving rise to the more complex multi layered epidermis seen in mature skin.

Q. 5. **Why do periderm cells undergo terminal differentiation to form a temporary protective layer during fetal development?**

Answer: Periderm cells undergo terminal differentiation to form a temporary protective layer during fetal development to because of following reason:
- Safeguard the underlying developing skin layers.
- This peridermal layer protects the fetal skin from
  - Mechanical damage and
  - Potential infections. It also
  - Prevents the loss of moisture.
- It eventually sheds and is replaced by the more permanent epidermal layers as the fetus matures.

Q. 6. **Why does epidermal atrophy lead to poor adhesion of the epidermis and its separation following minor injury?**

Answer: Epidermal atrophy leads to poor adhesion of the epidermis and its separation following minor injury because of following reason:
- General thinning and loss of the basal rete pegs,
- Flattening of the dermal-epidermal junction, and
- Decreased resistance to shear.

Q. 7. **Why is scar formation the end-point of healing of mammalian skin wounds?**

Answer: Scar formation is the end-point of healing of mammalian skin wounds because of following reason:
- Cutaneous scars result from injury to both
  - The epidermis and
  - The underlying dermis, and
  - The dermal architecture is abnormal after repair.

Q. 8. **Why do the cells of the deepest layer of the epidermis proliferate and migrate towards the surface?**

Answer: The cells of the deepest layer of the epidermis proliferate and migrate towards the surface because of following reason:
- This process continuously replaces the cornified cells lost due to wear and tear.
- It maintains the integrity and protective function of the skin by forming new layers of flattened, dead cells in the stratum corneum.

Dermal layer

Q. 9. **Why do the layers of the dermis provide mechanical anchorage and metabolic support to the epidermis?**

Answer: The layers of the dermis provide mechanical anchorage and metabolic support to the epidermis because of following reason:
- They contain a network of collagen and elastin fibers. It gives strength and flexibility to the skin. It helps to withstand physical stress.
- The dermis has blood vessels that supply nutrients and oxygen to the avascular epidermis.
- It ensures that its cells receive the necessary resources to function and regenerate.

Q. 10. **Why are melanocytes derived from the neural crest?**

Answer: Melanocytes are derived from the neural crest because of following reason:
- They originate from the neural crest cells during embryonic development.
- Neural crest cells are multipotent and migrate to various parts of the body, including the skin, where they differentiate into melanocytes.
- This migration and differentiation are crucial for the proper formation of pigment-producing cells. These are essential for skin color and UV protection.

Q. 11. **Why is the dermis derived from the somatopleuric mesenchyme and possibly the somatic mesenchyme?**

Answer: The dermis is derived from the somatopleuric mesenchyme and possibly the somatic mesenchyme because of following reason:
- These mesodermal layers provide the necessary connective tissue and structural support for skin development.
- Somatopleuric mesenchyme, associated with the body wall, contributes to the formation of the dermis's fibrous and vascular components.
- The somatic mesenchyme, associated with the body cavity linings, also supports the development of the dermal structure.
- These mesodermal origins ensure the proper formation and function of the dermal layer.

Q. 12. **Why do wrinkle lines become permanent with age as the skin loses its elasticity?**

Answer: Wrinkle lines become permanent with age because of following reason:
- The skin loses its elasticity due to a decrease in collagen and elastin production.
- As these supportive proteins diminish, the skin becomes less able to return to its original shape after stretching or movement.
- This results in the persistence of wrinkle lines, as the skin's ability to rebound and smooth out is reduced.

Q. 13. **Why do gradual changes occur in the appearance, microstructure, and mechanical properties of the skin from about the third decade onwards?**

Answer: Gradual changes in the appearance, microstructure, and mechanical properties of the skin from about the third decade onwards because of following reason:
- Occur due to aging.
- As people age, the skin undergoes a
    - Decrease in collagen and elastin production,
    - Reduced moisture retention, and
    - Slower cell turnover.
- These changes lead to
    - Thinning of the skin,
    - Reduced elasticity, and
    - Increased susceptibility to wrinkles and dryness.
- The cumulative effects of
    - Sun exposure,
    - Environmental factors, and
    - Natural aging processes contribute to these alterations.

Specialized skin areas (nails, hair, glands)

Q. 14. **Why do hair shafts consist of 3 concentric zones?**

Answer: Hair shafts consist of three concentric zones because of following reason:
The medulla,
- Cortex, and
- Cuticle—to provide structural strength and protection.
- The medulla, the innermost layer, adds thickness and strength.
- The cortex, which surrounds the medulla. It contains keratin and melanin, contributing to
    - The hair's texture and
    - Color. The cuticle, the outermost layer. It protects the inner layers from damage and helps retain moisture.

Q. 15. **Why are hair follicle stem cells found in the bulge regions below the sebaceous glands and in other parts of the hair follicle?**

Answer: Hair follicle stem cells are found in the bulge region below the sebaceous glands and in other parts of the hair follicle because of following reason:
- These locations provide a specialized microenvironment that
  - Protects and
  - Maintains the stem cells.
- The bulge region, in particular, offers
  - Signals and
  - Support that help these stem cells remain in a quiescent state until they are needed for
    - Hair growth,
    - Regeneration, or
    - Repair of the skin after injury.

Q. 16. **Why does the proximal part of the nail body present a white opaque crescent called the lunule?**

Answer: The proximal part of the nail body presents a white opaque crescent called the lunule because of following reason:
- This area is where the underlying germinative zone is thick and actively proliferating.
- It masks the underlying blood vessels and creates the distinct white appearance.

Q. 17. **Why does the skin beneath the root and body of the nail differ in thickness and function?**

Answer: The skin beneath the root and body of the nail differs in thickness and function because of following reason:
- The germinative zone beneath the root and lunule (germinal matrix) is thick and responsible for nail growth.
- The rest of the nail bed (sterile matrix) is thin and serves as a surface over which the nail glides as it grows.

Q. 18. **Why are the nails on the dorsal surface of the fingers and toes?**

Answer: Nails are on the dorsal surface of the fingers and toes because of following reason:
- This placement allows them to serve as
  - Protective and
  - Supportive structures for the tips of the digits.
- It helps in fine motor tasks and providing a barrier against injury.

Q. 19. **Why does the body of the nail appear pink under the translucent part?**
Answer: The body of the nail appears pink under the translucent part because of following reason:
- The corium (dermis) beneath the nail is highly vascular.
- The blood vessels present in this area give the nail its pink coloration through the translucent keratin plate.

Q. 20. **Why is the germinal matrix critical for nail growth?**
Answer: The germinal matrix is critical for nail growth because of following reason:
- It is the thick and proliferative part of the nail bed.
- Here new nail cells are produced.
- It, ensures continuous growth and regeneration of the nail plate.

Q. 21. **Why the scalp is considered the site with the maximum number of sebaceous glands?**
Answer: The scalp is considered the site with the maximum number of sebaceous glands because of following reason:
- It produces sebum to lubricate and protect the hair and skin.

Non-hairy skin

Q. 22. **Why are the palms, soles, dorsal surfaces of distal phalanges, umbilicus, glans penis, inner surface of the prepuce, inner surfaces of the labia majora, labia minora, surfaces of the eyelids, and exposed margins of the lips non-hairy surfaces of the body?**
Answer: The palms, soles, dorsal surfaces of distal phalanges, umbilicus, glans penis, inner surface of the prepuce, inner surfaces of the labia majora, labia minora, surfaces of the eyelids, and exposed margins of the lips are non-hairy surfaces of the body because of following reason:
- These areas serve specific functions that are better suited to being hairless:

Q. 23. **Why are the palms of the hands and soles of the feet considered the thickest skin in the body?**
Answer: The palms of the hands and soles of the feet are considered the thickest skin in the body because of following reason:
- They have a thick epidermal layer, particularly the stratum corneum.
- It is the outermost layer of the skin.
- This thickness provides
    - Protection against friction,
    - Pressure, and
    - Mechanical damage,

- These areas frequently encounter during activities like walking and gripping.
- Additionally, the skin in these areas lacks hair follicles and has a dense concentration of sweat glands, further contributing to its specialized structure and thickness.

Aging and skin function

Q. 24. Why is there a decrease in the sensitivity of sensory perception associated with ageing?

Answer: There is a decrease in the sensitivity of sensory perception associated with ageing because of following reason:
- Due to some loss of specialized receptors in the skin.

Q. 25. Why does photoageing occur as a result of the hazardous effect of UV radiation on human skin?

Answer: Photoageing occurs as a result of the hazardous effect of UV radiation on human skin because of following reason: It causes
- DNA damage,
- Angiogenesis,
- Lymphatic dysfunction, and
- The formation of reactive oxygen species, leading to skin ageing.

Q. 26. Why does the colour of the skin vary with the race, age, and part of the body?

Answer: The color of the skin varies with race, age, and part of the body due to several factors:
1. **Race**: Different races have varying levels of melanin, the pigment produced by melanocytes in the skin.
    - Higher melanin levels result in darker skin tones, while lower levels result in lighter skin.
    - Genetic differences influence melanin production, leading to the diversity of skin colors across races.
2. **Age**: As people age, skin color can change due to factors like
    - Reduced melanin production,
    - Thinning of the skin, and
    - Changes in blood flow.
    - Aging can also lead to the appearance of age spots and uneven pigmentation.
3. **Part of the body**: Skin color can vary on different parts of the body due to
    - Differences in sun exposure,
    - Thickness of the skin, and
    - The density of melanocytes.

- Areas that receive more sun exposure tend to have darker pigmentation as a protective response, while areas with thicker skin may appear lighter.

These factors combined lead to the variation in skin color observed across individuals and body parts.

Q. 27. Why do fair-skinned individuals have a higher risk of developing skin cancer?

Answer: Fair-skinned individuals have a higher risk of developing skin cancer because of following reason:
- They have less melanin, the pigment that protects the skin from ultraviolet (UV) radiation.
- Less melanin means less natural protection against UV damage.
- It increases the likelihood of DNA damage in skin cells and, consequently, a higher risk of skin cancer.

Development of skin

Q. 28. Why does the skin develop from the surface ectoderm and its underlying mesenchyme?

Answer: The skin develops from the surface ectoderm and its underlying mesenchyme because of following reason:
- These layers provide the necessary components for skin formation.
- The ectoderm gives rise to the epidermis.
- The mesenchyme, derived from mesoderm, forms the dermis.
- This interaction ensures the development of a functional skin layer with both
    - Protective and
    - Supportive roles.

Q. 29. Why are interactions between ectoderm and mesenchyme important in the development of the skin?

Answer: Interactions between ectoderm and mesenchyme are important in skin development because of following reason:
- They coordinate the formation and organization of the epidermis and dermis.
- The ectoderm differentiates into the epidermis.
- The mesenchyme, contributes to the dermis.
- It provides signals that regulate epidermal development. It contributes to the overall structure and function of the skin.
- This interaction ensures that both layers develop properly and work together to form a functional skin barrier.

Q. 30. **Why do externally visible skin lines increase the surface area of the skin?**

Answer: Externally visible skin lines, such as wrinkles and ridges because of following reason:
- Increase the surface area of the skin by folding or expanding the surface.
- These lines help accommodate changes in
    - Skin volume and
    - Movement.
- It provides flexibility and reduces mechanical stress.
- By increasing the surface area, the skin can better adapt to
    - Physical changes and
    - Maintain its protective functions.

Q. 31. **Why do papillary ridges form narrow parallel or curved arrays separated by narrow furrows?**

Answer: Papillary ridges form narrow parallel or curved arrays separated by narrow furrows because of following reason:
- To increase the skin's surface area and improve grip and friction.
- This arrangement enhances
    - The tactile sensitivity and
    - Grip of the skin by creating a more textured surface.
- The pattern also helps to anchor the epidermis more securely to the underlying dermis.
- It contributes to the overall stability and functionality of the skin.

Q. 32. **Why are Langer's Lines relevant in surgical incisions?**

Answer: Langer's Lines are relevant because surgical incisions because of following reason:
- Incisions made along these lines tend to heal better and with less scarring.
- It is due to the natural alignment of collagen fibers in the skin.
- Therefore it is a preferred approach for better cosmetic outcomes.

Skin healing and grafts

Q. 33. **Why are grafts pieces of tissue detached from their blood supply?**

Answer: Grafts are pieces of tissue detached from their blood supply because of following reason:
- They need to regain a blood supply from the bed in which they are placed in order to survive.

Q. 34. Why do full-thickness grafts tend to be taken from sites where the donor defect can be primarily closed?

Answer: Full-thickness grafts are taken from sites where the donor defect can be primarily closed to minimize the impact on the donor area.

- This approach ensures that the donor site heals effectively and reduces the risk of complications.
- By closing the defect primarily, the skin is restored more quickly and with less additional intervention
- It leads to a better overall outcome for both the donor and recipient sites.

Superficial fascia

Q. 35. Why does the superficial fascia allow mobility of the dermis on underlying structures?

Answer: The superficial fascia allows mobility of the dermis on underlying structures because of following reason:

- To facilitate movement and prevent restriction of skin movement.

Q. 36. Why the superficial fascia is heavily infiltrated with fat?

Answer: The superficial fascia is heavily infiltrated with fat because fat because of following reason:

- Serves as an insulating layer and provides cushioning at certain sites of the body.

Q. 37. Why does the amount of fat vary in different parts of the body's superficial fascia?

Answer: The amount of fat in different parts of the body's superficial fascia varies due to because of following reason:

- Differences in functional needs and genetic factors.
- For example, areas like the abdomen may store more fat for energy reserves and protection of internal organs, while other areas, such as the limbs, might have less fat due to different functional and structural requirements.
- Hormonal influences and individual variations also play a role in determining fat distribution.

Q. 38. **Why is the superficial fascia responsible for the smooth external contours of females?**

Answer: The superficial fascia is responsible for the smooth external contours of females because of following reason:
- It contains a higher amount of fat deposits compared to males.
- These fat deposits fill out the spaces under the skin, creating smooth and rounded contours, especially in areas like
    - The hips,
    - Thighs, and
    - Breasts.
- This distribution of fat is influenced by hormones like estrogen, giving females their characteristic body shape.

Q. 39. **Why does the superficial fascia act as a distributing layer for blood vessels, lymphatics, and nerves?**

Answer: The superficial fascia acts as a distributing layer for blood vessels, lymphatics, and nerves because of following reason:
- It lies just beneath the skin and serves as a connective tissue layer that supports.
- It separates the skin from the underlying muscles and structures.
- This fascia provides a flexible and cushioning environment that allows these structures to branch out and distribute throughout the body.
- It ensures that
    - Blood vessels,
    - Lymphatics, and
    - Nerves can reach the skin and other superficial tissues, while also providing protection and insulation.

Q. 40. **Why does the superficial fascia act as a cushion at certain sites of the body?**

Answer: The superficial fascia acts as a cushion at certain sites of the body because of following reason:
- It contains a layer of fat that provides padding and absorbs shock.
- This fat helps protect underlying structures, such as
    - Muscles,
    - Bones, and
    - Organs, from external pressure and impact.
- In areas like the buttocks, palms, and soles of the feet, the thicker layer of fat in the superficial fascia offers extra cushioning to support and protect these regions from frequent pressure and stress.

Q. 41. **Why does superficial fascia facilitate movements of the skin?**
Answer: Superficial fascia facilitates movements of the skin because of following reason:
- It provides a flexible medium through which the skin can slide over underlying structures.

Q. 42. **Why is fat more abundant and evenly distributed in females than in males?**
Answer: Fat is more abundant and evenly distributed in females than in males because of following reason:
- It serves as an energy reserve and contributes to reproductive functions.

Q. 43. **Why does superficial fascia conserve body heat?**
Answer: Superficial fascia conserves body heat because of following reason:
- It contains a layer of adipose (fat) tissue.
- This fat acts as an insulator, reducing heat loss from the body by trapping warm air and preventing it from escaping.

Q. 44. **Why are superficial fascia and fat most distinct in the lower part of the anterior abdominal wall?**
Answer: Superficial fascia and fat are most distinct in the lower part of the anterior abdominal wall because of following reason:
- This area is adapted to store more fat. The fat serves as an energy reserve and provides insulation.
- Additionally, the lower abdomen is more prone to fat accumulation due to hormonal and genetic factors.

Q. 45. **Why does fat fill hollow spaces like the axilla and ischiorectal fossa?**
Answer: Fat fills hollow spaces like the axilla and ischiorectal fossa to provide cushioning and support because of following reason:
- It helps
  - Stabilize and protect underlying structures,
  - Absorbs shocks, and
  - Allows for smooth movement of adjacent tissues.

Deep fascia

Q. 46. Why is the deep fascia described as a tough, inelastic membrane of fibrous tissue?

Answer: The deep fascia is described as a tough, inelastic membrane of fibrous tissue because of following reason:
- It is composed primarily of dense connective tissue with tightly packed collagen fibers.
- These collagen fibers give the deep fascia its strength and durability, making it resistant to stretching and deformation.
- This inelasticity helps the deep fascia maintain the structural integrity of
    - Muscles,
    - Bones, and
    - Other underlying tissues, providing
        - Support,
        - Protection, and
        - Compartmentalization within the body.

Q. 47. Why does the deep fascia send septa between groups of muscles in the limbs?

Answer: The deep fascia sends septa between groups of muscles in the limbs because of following reason:
- To attach with the periosteum of the bone.
- It allows individual muscle groups to contract independently.
- It slides freely over adjacent muscles.

Q. 48. Why does the deep fascia form 3 layers in the neck?

Answer: The deep fascia forms three layers in the neck because of following reason:
- To organize and compartmentalize the various structures within the neck, providing support and protection. These layers are:
1. **Investing layer:** this outermost layer surrounds the entire neck, enclosing muscles like the sternocleidomastoid and trapezius, and helping to define the neck's shape.
2. **Pretracheal layer:** this middle layer surrounds the trachea, esophagus, and thyroid gland, providing a protective compartment for these vital structures.
3. **Prevertebral layer:** this innermost layer covers the vertebral column and associated muscles, offering additional support and stability to the spine.

By forming these distinct layers, the deep fascia ensures that the different structures in the neck are securely held in place, allowing for efficient movement and function while protecting them from injury.

Q. 49. **Why does the deep fascia attach to bone wherever it encounters it?**
Answer: The deep fascia attaches to bone wherever it encounters it to provide stability and anchorage for muscles and other structures. This attachment helps
- To transmit the force generated by muscles during movement.
- It ensures that the muscles can effectively exert their action on the bones.
- By anchoring to the bone, the deep fascia also helps to compartmentalize muscles.
- It prevents excessive movement of tissues, maintaining the organization and functional integrity of the musculoskeletal system.

Q. 50. **Why does the deep fascia form retinacula at certain sites?**
Answer: The deep fascia forms retinacula at certain sites
- To hold tendons in place as they pass over joints.
- Retinacula are thickened bands of fascia that prevent the tendons from bowing outward when muscles contract, ensuring that the tendons remain close to the bones.
- This arrangement allows for efficient transmission of force from the muscles to the bones, contributing to precise and controlled movements.
- Retinacula are especially important in areas like the wrist and ankle, where multiple tendons pass over joints and need to be stabilized.

Q. 51. **Why does the deep fascia thicken to form aponeurosis in palms and soles?**
Answer: The deep fascia thickens to form aponeuroses in the palms and soles
- To provide
    - Strength,
    - Stability, and
    - Protection in these areas that experience frequent stress and pressure.
- These thickened sheets of fibrous tissue help distribute the forces exerted on the hands and feet during activities like
    - Gripping,
    - Walking, and
    - Running.
- In the palms, the palmar aponeurosis supports the skin and underlying structures, enhancing grip and preventing slippage.
- In the soles, the plantar aponeurosis helps maintain the arches of the foot, providing support and shock absorption.

Q. 52. **Why does the deep fascia condense to form fibrous sheaths around neurovascular bundles?**

Answer: The deep fascia condenses to form fibrous sheaths around neurovascular bundles of following reason:
- Such as the carotid sheath and axillary sheath, to provide
    - Structural support and
    - Protection while allowing veins to distend.

Q. 53. **Why does the deep fascia split to enclose certain glands?**

Answer: The deep fascia splits to enclose certain glands of following reason:
- Fibrous capsules, such as the parotid gland and submandibular gland, to
    - Protect and
    - Support these structures.

Q. 54. **Why is the deep fascia modified to form interosseous membranes in the forearm and leg?**

Answer: The deep fascia is modified to form interosseous membranes in the forearm and leg of following reason:
- To bind adjacent bones together and
- Maintain their alignment.

Q. 55. **Why does the deep fascia send intermuscular septa in the limbs?**

Answer: The deep fascia sends intermuscular septa in the limbs of following reason:
- To help form compartments for muscles. ,
- It allows groups of muscles to function independently.

Q. 56. **Why does the deep fascia thicken to form fibrous flexor sheaths on the flexor surfaces of fingers and toes?**

Answer: The deep fascia thickens to form fibrous flexor sheaths on the flexor surfaces of fingers and toes of following reason:
- To prevent long flexor tendons from bowing out of position during movement.

Q. 57. **Why are ligaments considered as localized thickened bands of the deep fascia?**

Answer: Ligaments are considered as localized thickened bands of the deep fascia because of following reason:
- They provide additional support and stability to joints,
- They function similarly to the deep fascia in other areas of the body.

Q. 58. **Why does the deep fascia form fascial sheaths around certain muscles, such as the psoas sheath?**

Answer: The deep fascia forms fascial sheaths around certain muscles,
- Such as the psoas sheath, to provide
    - Support,
    - Protection, and
    - Facilitate smooth movement.
- These sheaths encase the muscles, helping to maintain their shape and alignment during contraction and relaxation.
- The fascial sheath also reduces friction between the muscle and surrounding tissues, allowing for efficient movement.
- Additionally, by compartmentalising the muscles, the fascial sheath can help contain the spread of infections or inflammation. It provides an added layer of protection to the body.

Q. 59. **Why is the deep fascia absent at certain sites, such as the face and breast?**

Answer: The deep fascia is absent at certain sites, such as the face and breast,
- To allow for
    - Greater flexibility,
    - Movement, and
    - Accommodation of underlying structures.
- In the face, the absence of deep fascia allows for a wide range of facial expressions by providing the muscles of facial expression the freedom to move the overlying skin directly.
- In the breast, the lack of deep fascia allows
    - The breast tissue to expand and
    - Change shape, which is important for functions like
        - Breastfeeding and
        - Responding to hormonal changes.
- Additionally, the absence of deep fascia in these areas permits a softer and more pliable texture, which is important for the aesthetic and functional characteristics of these regions.

Q. 60. **Why is the deep fascia very sensitive?**
Answer: The deep fascia is very sensitive because
- It contains a network of nerve endings, including those that detect
    - Pain,
    - Pressure, and
    - Stretch.
- This sensitivity allows the deep fascia to respond to
    - Mechanical changes and
    - Potential injuries.
- It plays a role in proprioception, helping the body sense and adjust to changes in muscle tension and movement.
- Additionally, the sensitivity of the deep fascia helps protect underlying structures by alerting the body to potential harm or excessive strain.

Q. 61. **Why does the deep fascia facilitate venous and lymphatic drainage?**
Answer: The deep fascia facilitates venous and lymphatic drainage because of following reason:
- By providing
    - Pathways and
    - Support structures for these systems.

Q. 62. **Why does the deep fascia retain long tendons in place?**
Answer: The deep fascia retains long tendons in place because of following reason:
- To prevent their bowstringing during muscle action.
- It serves as pulleys to enhance their efficiency.

Q. 63. **Why does deep fascia help in venous and lymphatic return from the lower limb?**
Answer: Deep fascia helps in venous and lymphatic return from the lower limb by
- Creating a pressure gradient that assists blood and lymph flow.
- It tightly encases muscles, which contract during movement, compressing veins and lymphatic vessels.
- It facilitates the return of blood and lymph toward the heart.

Q. 64. **Why is deep fascia important for maintaining the surface contour of the limbs and neck?**
Answer: Deep fascia is important for maintaining the surface contour of the limbs and neck because of following reason:
- It keeps underlying structures in position and supports the characteristic appearance of these body parts.

Q. 65. **Why are retinacula important in the limbs?**

Answer: Retinacula are important in the limbs because
- They act as strong bands of connective tissue that hold tendons in place during movement.
- This prevents the tendons from slipping out of their proper positions, ensuring efficient and controlled movement of the joints and muscles.

Q. 66. **Why does deep fascia form fibroareolar sheaths around muscles, vessels, and nerves?**

Answer: Deep fascia forms fibroareolar sheaths around muscles, vessels, and nerves because of following reason:
- To provide support and protection to these structures within the compartments of the body.

Q. 67. **Why does deep fascia form interosseous membranes in the forearm and leg?**

Answer: Deep fascia forms interosseous membranes in the forearm and leg because of following reason:
- To keep bones at an optimum distance, increase the surface area for muscle attachment, and transmit weight from one bone to another.

Miscellaneous questions

Q. 68. **Why are flexure (joint) lines major markings found in the vicinity of synovial joints?**

Answer: Flexure (joint) lines are major markings found in the vicinity of synovial joints because of following reason:
- They accommodate the skin's movement and folding at these areas of frequent bending.
- These lines help the skin to
    - Flex and
    - Stretch more effectively around the joints.
- It prevents stress and damage to the skin as it moves with the underlying joints and muscles.

Q. 69. **Why does wound healing often involve the coordination of numerous cell types, signalling molecules, and matrix proteins**

Answer: Wound healing often involves the coordination of numerous cell types, signalling molecules, and matrix proteins because of following reason:
- The complex balance of these mediators, rather than their individual action, determines events in wound repair.

Q. 70. **Why is wound contraction an important part of remodelling in wound healing?**

Answer: Wound contraction is an important part of remodelling in wound healing because of following reason:
- Myofibroblasts generated from activated fibroblasts play a key role in pulling normal dermal and adipose tissue.
- They migrate into the wound defect.
- They help to scar formation.

Q. 71. **Why does revascularization of grafts depend on early and direct connection between host and graft vessels?**

Answer: Revascularization of grafts depends on early and direct connection between host and graft vessels because of following reason:
- This connection is crucial for restoring blood supply to the graft.
- The graft needs an adequate blood supply to receive oxygen and nutrients and to remove waste products.
- Early and direct vascular connection helps to ensure the graft survives. It integrates with the surrounding tissue.
- It reduces the risk of graft failure and promoting successful healing.

Q. 72. **Why does the skin contain stem cells in various parts of the hair follicles, basal layer of the interfollicular epidermis, and within sweat glands?**

Answer: The skin contains stem cells in various parts, such as
- Hair follicles,
- The basal layer of the interfollicular epidermis, and
- Within sweat glands, because
- These cells are crucial for
    - Tissue repair and
    - Regeneration.
- When the skin is damage, these stem cells can divide and differentiate into various cell types needed to heal wounds and maintain the skin's integrity.

Q. 73. **Why is the skin regarded as an important organ of the body?**

Answer: The skin is regarded as an important organ of the body because of following reason:
- It performs a large number of essential functions, including
    - Protection,
    - Sensation,
    - Temperature regulation, and
    - Synthesis of vitamin D, making it crucial for overall health and homeostasis.

Q. 74. **Why does the colour of the skin depend on the vascularity of the dermis and the thickness of the keratin in white races?**

Answer: The color of the skin in white races depends on the vascularity of the dermis and the thickness of the keratin because of following reason:
- These factors influence how light is absorbed and reflected by the skin.
- **Vascularity of the dermis**: Blood vessels in the dermis can give the skin a pinkish or reddish hue depending on the amount of blood flow.
    - This effect is more noticeable in people with lighter skin, where the underlying blood vessels are more visible.
- **Thickness of the keratin**: The thickness of the keratin layer in the epidermis can affect how much of this underlying color is visible.
    - Thicker keratin can make the skin appear paler, as it blocks some of the color from the blood vessels.

Together, these factors contribute to the overall color of the skin

Q. 75. **Why does the thickness of the skin vary from about 0.5 to 3 mm?**

Answer: The thickness of the skin varies from about 0.5 to 3 mm because of following reason:
- Different body areas require different levels of protection and flexibility.
- Thicker skin, such as on the palms and soles, provides greater protection and durability,
- Thinner skin in other areas allows for greater sensitivity and flexibility.

Q. 76. Why does the skin have surface irregularities like tension lines, flexure lines, and papillary ridges?

Answer: The skin has surface irregularities like tension lines, flexure lines, and papillary ridges because of following reason:
- These features help
    - Accommodate movement,
    - Improve grip, and
    - Enhance the skin's ability to
        - Stretch and
        - Return to its original shape.
- Tension lines correspond to underlying fiber patterns.
- , Flexure lines occur at joints, and papillary ridges provide friction ridges for better tactile sensation and grip.

Q. 77. Why do the epidermis of the skin, hair, nails, cornea of the eye, lens, articular hyaline cartilages, splenic pulp, brain and spinal cord, and bone marrow lack blood capillaries?

Answer: The epidermis of the skin, hair, nails, cornea of the eye, lens, articular hyaline cartilage, splenic pulp, brain and spinal cord, and bone marrow lack blood capillaries because they are either avascular tissues or specialized regions where direct blood supply could interfere with their function.

1. **Epidermis of the skin, hair, and nails**: These tissues are avascular, meaning they do not have blood vessels.
   - Nutrients and oxygen are supplied through diffusion from the underlying dermis.
   - This arrangement helps protect against injury and infection, as it limits direct access to the bloodstream.
2. **Cornea and lens of the eye**: These structures need to be transparent to allow light to pass through for vision.
   - Blood vessels would obstruct this transparency.
   - They rely on diffusion of nutrients from surrounding fluids, like the aqueous humor.
3. **Articular hyaline cartilage**: This cartilage covers the ends of bones in joints.
   - **It** must be smooth and resilient to reduce friction and absorb shock.
   - Blood vessels would interfere with these mechanical properties.
   - So the cartilage is nourished by synovial fluid in the joint.
4. **Splenic pulp**: The splenic pulp consists mainly of red and white pulp.
   - It filters blood and produce immune responses.
   - The spleen is highly vascularized
   - The specific tissue arrangement avoids direct blood capillaries within the pulp to facilitate its filtering and immune functions.
5. **Brain and spinal cord**: These structures are protected by the blood-brain barrier.

- **It** regulates the passage of substances from the blood to the nervous tissue.
- Capillaries in the brain and spinal cord have special properties that maintain this barrier.
- It reduces the risk of harmful substances entering the nervous system.

6. **Bone marrow**: Bone marrow is highly vascularized overall, but the areas where blood cell production occurs are separated from the capillaries by a specialized structure.
   - This allows for the controlled release of new blood cells into circulation.

In all these cases, the lack of direct blood capillaries is an adaptation to preserve the function and integrity of the tissue or organ.

Q. 78. Why the labia minora are termed sex skin?

Answer: The labia minora are termed "sex skin" because of following reason:
- They are sensitive to hormonal changes and respond to sexual stimulation.
- These inner folds of the vulva are rich in blood vessels and nerve endings, making them highly responsive to sexual arousal.
- During sexual activity, the labia minora can swell and change color due to increased blood flow, which is why they are referred to as "sex skin."

Q. 79. Why the face is considered the commonest site of skin cancer?

Answer: The face is considered the commonest site of skin cancer because of following reason:
- It is frequently exposed to ultraviolet (UV) radiation from the sun.
- The skin on the face is often unprotected, making it more vulnerable to the damaging effects of UV rays.
- It can cause mutations in skin cells and lead to the development of cancer.
- Additionally, the face has a high density of skin cells that are prone to cancer, such as basal and squamous cells, increasing the risk of skin cancer in this area.

Q. 80. Why moles are considered the commonest congenital disorder of the skin?

Answer: Moles are considered the most common congenital disorder of the skin because of following reason:
- They often appear as harmless pigmented spots or growths at birth or develop shortly after.
- They result from an overgrowth of melanocytes,
- Melanocytes are responsible for pigment in the skin.
- While most moles are benign, their prevalence and ease of detection make them a common example of skin disorders that people are born with or acquire early in life.

Q. 81. **Why the mammary gland is considered the largest modified gland of the skin in females?**

Answer: The mammary gland is considered the largest modified gland of the skin in females because of following reason:
- It originates from the skin's sweat glands and undergoes significant development.
- It is large compared to other skin glands due to its role in producing milk, which involves complex structures and extensive tissue growth.
- This functional adaptation makes it notably larger and more specialized than other modified skin glands.

Q. 82. **Why Pacinian corpuscles are considered the largest sensory receptors of the skin?**

Answer: Pacinian corpuscles are considered the largest sensory receptors of the skin because of following reason:
- They detect deep pressure and vibration, located in the deeper layers of the skin.

Q. 83. **Why a lipoma is considered the most common tumor arising from subcutaneous tissue?**

Answer: A lipoma is considered the most common tumor arising from subcutaneous tissue Because of following reason:
- It is a benign growth of fatty tissue that frequently occurs under the skin.

Q. 84. **Why is the Malpighian layer significant in dermatology?**

Answer: The Malpighian layer, or germinative layer of the epidermis, is significant because of following reason:
- It is the site of cell division and the generation of new skin cells.
- It indicates its importance in skin regeneration and repair.

Q. 85. **Why do wounds of the skin heal quickly?**

Answer: Wounds of the skin heal quickly due to because of following reason:
- The skin's ability to regenerate and repair itself.
- The skin has a rich supply of blood vessels that deliver nutrients and oxygen essential for healing.
- Additionally, the skin's cells proliferate rapidly to cover the wound, and various growth factors and immune cells help manage inflammation and prevent infection.

Q. 86. **Why is skin cancer most often associated with the face and neck regions?**

Answer: Skin cancer is most often associated with the face and neck regions because of following reason:
- These areas are usually not covered, making them more exposed to ultraviolet radiation from the sun.

Q. 87. **Why do incisions made parallel to cleavage lines result in less unsightly scars?**

Answer: Incisions made parallel to cleavage lines result in less unsightly scars because of following reason:
- They sever fewer collagen fibers.
- They have decrease tendency of the fibers to retract and resulting in a finer, hairline scar.

7. Skin and fascia

Epidermal layer (keratinocytes, melanocytes, merkel cells)

Q. 88. **Why do melanocytes produce melanin pigment?**
Answer: Melanocytes produce melanin pigment because of following reason:
- To protect the skin from the harmful effects of ultraviolet (UV) radiation.
- Melanin absorbs and disperses UV rays, reducing the risk of DNA damage in skin cells.
- It helps to prevent skin cancer.
- It also gives color to the skin, hair, and eyes.

Q. 89. **Why do ectodermal cells differentiate mainly into keratinocytes and probably Merkel cells?**
Answer: Ectodermal cells differentiate mainly into keratinocytes and Merkel cells because of following reason:
- These cell types are essential for the skin's functions.
- Keratinocytes form the primary protective layer of the epidermis. It produces keratin that
    - Strengthens and
    - Protects the skin.
- Merkel cells, although less abundant. They are involved in sensory functions, specifically touch and pressure sensation.
- This differentiation is crucial for the skin's role in protection, sensation, and maintaining homeostasis.

Q. 90. **Why do nerves and associated Schwann cells enter and traverse the dermis during development?**
Answer: Nerves and associated Schwann cells enter and traverse the dermis during development because of following reason:
- To establish the sensory and autonomic nerve networks necessary for skin function.
- Schwann cells provide support and insulation to nerve fibers, facilitating efficient signal transmission.
- This network allows the skin to detect and respond to various stimuli, such as touch, temperature, and pain, and plays a role in regulating blood flow and other skin functions.

Q. 91. **Why does the epidermis develop into a bilaminar epithelium during embryonic development?**

Answer: The epidermis develops into a bilaminar epithelium during embryonic development to because of following reason:
- Establish 2 distinct layers:
    - The periderm and
    - The basal layer.
- The periderm acts as a temporary protective layer, while the basal layer forms the foundation for the future stratified epidermis.
- This bilaminar structure is crucial for initial skin formation and protection as the fetus develops, eventually giving rise to the more complex multi layered epidermis seen in mature skin.

Q. 92. **Why do periderm cells undergo terminal differentiation to form a temporary protective layer during fetal development?**

Answer: Periderm cells undergo terminal differentiation to form a temporary protective layer during fetal development to because of following reason:
- Safeguard the underlying developing skin layers.
- This peridermal layer protects the fetal skin from
    - Mechanical damage and
    - Potential infections. It also
    - Prevents the loss of moisture.
- It eventually sheds and is replaced by the more permanent epidermal layers as the fetus matures.

Q. 93. **Why does epidermal atrophy lead to poor adhesion of the epidermis and its separation following minor injury?**

Answer: Epidermal atrophy leads to poor adhesion of the epidermis and its separation following minor injury because of following reason:
- General thinning and loss of the basal rete pegs,
- Flattening of the dermal-epidermal junction, and
- Decreased resistance to shear.

Q. 94. **Why is scar formation the end-point of healing of mammalian skin wounds?**

Answer: Scar formation is the end-point of healing of mammalian skin wounds because of following reason:
- Cutaneous scars result from injury to both
    - The epidermis and
    - The underlying dermis, and
    - The dermal architecture is abnormal after repair.

Q. 95. **Why do the cells of the deepest layer of the epidermis proliferate and migrate towards the surface?**

Answer: The cells of the deepest layer of the epidermis proliferate and migrate towards the surface because of following reason:
- This process continuously replaces the cornified cells lost due to wear and tear.
- It maintains the integrity and protective function of the skin by forming new layers of flattened, dead cells in the stratum corneum.

Dermal layer

Q. 96. **Why do the layers of the dermis provide mechanical anchorage and metabolic support to the epidermis?**

Answer: The layers of the dermis provide mechanical anchorage and metabolic support to the epidermis because of following reason:
- They contain a network of collagen and elastin fibers. It gives strength and flexibility to the skin. It helps to withstand physical stress.
- The dermis has blood vessels that supply nutrients and oxygen to the avascular epidermis.
- It ensures that its cells receive the necessary resources to function and regenerate.

Q. 97. **Why are melanocytes derived from the neural crest?**

Answer: Melanocytes are derived from the neural crest because of following reason:
- They originate from the neural crest cells during embryonic development.
- Neural crest cells are multipotent and migrate to various parts of the body, including the skin, where they differentiate into melanocytes.
- This migration and differentiation are crucial for the proper formation of pigment-producing cells. These are essential for skin color and UV protection.

Q. 98. **Why is the dermis derived from the somatopleuric mesenchyme and possibly the somatic mesenchyme?**

Answer: The dermis is derived from the somatopleuric mesenchyme and possibly the somatic mesenchyme because of following reason:
- These mesodermal layers provide the necessary connective tissue and structural support for skin development.
- Somatopleuric mesenchyme, associated with the body wall, contributes to the formation of the dermis's fibrous and vascular components.
- The somatic mesenchyme, associated with the body cavity linings, also supports the development of the dermal structure.
- These mesodermal origins ensure the proper formation and function of the dermal layer.

Q. 99. **Why do wrinkle lines become permanent with age as the skin loses its elasticity?**

Answer: Wrinkle lines become permanent with age because of following reason:
- The skin loses its elasticity due to a decrease in collagen and elastin production.
- As these supportive proteins diminish, the skin becomes less able to return to its original shape after stretching or movement.
- This results in the persistence of wrinkle lines, as the skin's ability to rebound and smooth out is reduced.

Q. 100. **Why do gradual changes occur in the appearance, microstructure, and mechanical properties of the skin from about the third decade onwards?**

Answer: Gradual changes in the appearance, microstructure, and mechanical properties of the skin from about the third decade onwards because of following reason:
- Occur due to aging.
- As people age, the skin undergoes a
    - Decrease in collagen and elastin production,
    - Reduced moisture retention, and
    - Slower cell turnover.
- These changes lead to
    - Thinning of the skin,
    - Reduced elasticity, and
    - Increased susceptibility to wrinkles and dryness.
- The cumulative effects of
    - Sun exposure,
    - Environmental factors, and
    - Natural aging processes contribute to these alterations.

Specialized skin areas (nails, hair, glands)

Q. 101. **Why do hair shafts consist of 3 concentric zones?**

Answer: Hair shafts consist of three concentric zones because of following reason:
The medulla,
- Cortex, and
- Cuticle — to provide structural strength and protection.
- The medulla, the innermost layer, adds thickness and strength.
- The cortex, which surrounds the medulla. It contains keratin and melanin, contributing to
    - The hair's texture and
    - Color. The cuticle, the outermost layer. It protects the inner layers from damage and helps retain moisture.

Q. 102. **Why are hair follicle stem cells found in the bulge regions below the sebaceous glands and in other parts of the hair follicle?**

Answer: Hair follicle stem cells are found in the bulge region below the sebaceous glands and in other parts of the hair follicle because of following reason:
- These locations provide a specialized microenvironment that
    - Protects and
    - Maintains the stem cells.
- The bulge region, in particular, offers
    - Signals and
    - Support that help these stem cells remain in a quiescent state until they are needed for
        - Hair growth,
        - Regeneration, or
        - Repair of the skin after injury.

Q. 103. **Why does the proximal part of the nail body present a white opaque crescent called the lunule?**

Answer: The proximal part of the nail body presents a white opaque crescent called the lunule because of following reason:
- This area is where the underlying germinative zone is thick and actively proliferating.
- It masks the underlying blood vessels and creates the distinct white appearance.

Q. 104. **Why does the skin beneath the root and body of the nail differ in thickness and function?**

Answer: The skin beneath the root and body of the nail differs in thickness and function because of following reason:
- The germinative zone beneath the root and lunule (germinal matrix) is thick and responsible for nail growth.
- The rest of the nail bed (sterile matrix) is thin and serves as a surface over which the nail glides as it grows.

Q. 105. **Why are the nails on the dorsal surface of the fingers and toes?**

Answer: Nails are on the dorsal surface of the fingers and toes because of following reason:
- This placement allows them to serve as
    - Protective and
    - Supportive structures for the tips of the digits.
- It helps in fine motor tasks and providing a barrier against injury.

Q. 106. **Why does the body of the nail appear pink under the translucent part?**
Answer: The body of the nail appears pink under the translucent part because of following reason:
- The corium (dermis) beneath the nail is highly vascular.
- The blood vessels present in this area give the nail its pink coloration through the translucent keratin plate.

Q. 107. **Why is the germinal matrix critical for nail growth?**
Answer: The germinal matrix is critical for nail growth because of following reason:
- It is the thick and proliferative part of the nail bed.
- Here new nail cells are produced.
- It, ensures continuous growth and regeneration of the nail plate.

Q. 108. **Why the scalp is considered the site with the maximum number of sebaceous glands?**
Answer: The scalp is considered the site with the maximum number of sebaceous glands because of following reason:
- It produces sebum to lubricate and protect the hair and skin.

Non-hairy skin

Q. 109. **Why are the palms, soles, dorsal surfaces of distal phalanges, umbilicus, glans penis, inner surface of the prepuce, inner surfaces of the labia majora, labia minora, surfaces of the eyelids, and exposed margins of the lips non-hairy surfaces of the body?**

Answer: The palms, soles, dorsal surfaces of distal phalanges, umbilicus, glans penis, inner surface of the prepuce, inner surfaces of the labia majora, labia minora, surfaces of the eyelids, and exposed margins of the lips are non-hairy surfaces of the body because of following reason:

- These areas serve specific functions that are better suited to being hairless:

Q. 110. **Why are the palms of the hands and soles of the feet considered the thickest skin in the body?**
Answer: The palms of the hands and soles of the feet are considered the thickest skin in the body because of following reason:
- They have a thick epidermal layer, particularly the stratum corneum.
- It is the outermost layer of the skin.
- This thickness provides
    - Protection against friction,
    - Pressure, and

- o Mechanical damage,
- These areas frequently encounter during activities like walking and gripping.
- Additionally, the skin in these areas lacks hair follicles and has a dense concentration of sweat glands, further contributing to its specialized structure and thickness.

Aging and skin function

Q. 111. Why is there a decrease in the sensitivity of sensory perception associated with ageing?

Answer: There is a decrease in the sensitivity of sensory perception associated with ageing because of following reason:
- Due to some loss of specialized receptors in the skin.

Q. 112. Why does photoageing occur as a result of the hazardous effect of UV radiation on human skin?

Answer: Photoageing occurs as a result of the hazardous effect of UV radiation on human skin because of following reason: It causes
- DNA damage,
- Angiogenesis,
- Lymphatic dysfunction, and
- The formation of reactive oxygen species, leading to skin ageing.

Q. 113. Why does the colour of the skin vary with the race, age, and part of the body?

Answer: The color of the skin varies with race, age, and part of the body due to several factors:

4. **Race**: Different races have varying levels of melanin, the pigment produced by melanocytes in the skin.
   - Higher melanin levels result in darker skin tones, while lower levels result in lighter skin.
   - Genetic differences influence melanin production, leading to the diversity of skin colors across races.
5. **Age**: As people age, skin color can change due to factors like
   - Reduced melanin production,
   - Thinning of the skin, and
   - Changes in blood flow.
   - Aging can also lead to the appearance of age spots and uneven pigmentation.
6. **Part of the body**: Skin color can vary on different parts of the body due to
   - Differences in sun exposure,

- Thickness of the skin, and
- The density of melanocytes.
- Areas that receive more sun exposure tend to have darker pigmentation as a protective response, while areas with thicker skin may appear lighter.

These factors combined lead to the variation in skin color observed across individuals and body parts.

Q. 114. **Why do fair-skinned individuals have a higher risk of developing skin cancer?**

Answer: Fair-skinned individuals have a higher risk of developing skin cancer because of following reason:
- They have less melanin, the pigment that protects the skin from ultraviolet (UV) radiation.
- Less melanin means less natural protection against UV damage.
- It increases the likelihood of DNA damage in skin cells and, consequently, a higher risk of skin cancer.

Development of skin

Q. 115. **Why does the skin develop from the surface ectoderm and its underlying mesenchyme?**

Answer: The skin develops from the surface ectoderm and its underlying mesenchyme because of following reason:
- These layers provide the necessary components for skin formation.
- The ectoderm gives rise to the epidermis.
- The mesenchyme, derived from mesoderm, forms the dermis.
- This interaction ensures the development of a functional skin layer with both
    o Protective and
    o Supportive roles.

Q. 116. **Why are interactions between ectoderm and mesenchyme important in the development of the skin?**

Answer: Interactions between ectoderm and mesenchyme are important in skin development because of following reason:
- They coordinate the formation and organization of the epidermis and dermis.
- The ectoderm differentiates into the epidermis.
- The mesenchyme, contributes to the dermis.
- It provides signals that regulate epidermal development. It contributes to the overall structure and function of the skin.
- This interaction ensures that both layers develop properly and work together to form a functional skin barrier.

Q. 117. **Why do externally visible skin lines increase the surface area of the skin?**

Answer: Externally visible skin lines, such as wrinkles and ridges because of following reason:
- Increase the surface area of the skin by folding or expanding the surface.
- These lines help accommodate changes in
    - Skin volume and
    - Movement.
- It provides flexibility and reduces mechanical stress.
- By increasing the surface area, the skin can better adapt to
    - Physical changes and
    - Maintain its protective functions.

Q. 118. **Why do papillary ridges form narrow parallel or curved arrays separated by narrow furrows?**

Answer: Papillary ridges form narrow parallel or curved arrays separated by narrow furrows because of following reason:
- To increase the skin's surface area and improve grip and friction.
- This arrangement enhances
    - The tactile sensitivity and
    - Grip of the skin by creating a more textured surface.
- The pattern also helps to anchor the epidermis more securely to the underlying dermis.
- It contributes to the overall stability and functionality of the skin.

Q. 119. **Why are Langer's Lines relevant in surgical incisions?**

Answer: Langer's Lines are relevant because surgical incisions because of following reason:
- Incisions made along these lines tend to heal better and with less scarring.
- It is due to the natural alignment of collagen fibers in the skin.
- Therefore it is a preferred approach for better cosmetic outcomes.

Skin healing and grafts

Q. 120. **Why are grafts pieces of tissue detached from their blood supply?**

Answer: Grafts are pieces of tissue detached from their blood supply because of following reason:
- They need to regain a blood supply from the bed in which they are placed in order to survive.

Q. 121. **Why do full-thickness grafts tend to be taken from sites where the donor defect can be primarily closed?**

Answer: Full-thickness grafts are taken from sites where the donor defect can be primarily closed to minimize the impact on the donor area.
- This approach ensures that the donor site heals effectively and reduces the risk of complications.
- By closing the defect primarily, the skin is restored more quickly and with less additional intervention
- It leads to a better overall outcome for both the donor and recipient sites.

Superficial fascia

Q. 122. **Why does the superficial fascia allow mobility of the dermis on underlying structures?**

Answer: The superficial fascia allows mobility of the dermis on underlying structures because of following reason:
- To facilitate movement and prevent restriction of skin movement.

Q. 123. **Why the superficial fascia is heavily infiltrated with fat?**

Answer: The superficial fascia is heavily infiltrated with fat because fat because of following reason:
- Serves as an insulating layer and provides cushioning at certain sites of the body.

Q. 124. **Why does the amount of fat vary in different parts of the body's superficial fascia?**

Answer: The amount of fat in different parts of the body's superficial fascia varies due to because of following reason:
- Differences in functional needs and genetic factors.
- For example, areas like the abdomen may store more fat for energy reserves and protection of internal organs, while other areas, such as the limbs, might have less fat due to different functional and structural requirements.
- Hormonal influences and individual variations also play a role in determining fat distribution.

Q. 125. **Why is the superficial fascia responsible for the smooth external contours of females?**

Answer: The superficial fascia is responsible for the smooth external contours of females because of following reason:
- It contains a higher amount of fat deposits compared to males.
- These fat deposits fill out the spaces under the skin, creating smooth and rounded contours, especially in areas like
    - The hips,
    - Thighs, and
    - Breasts.
- This distribution of fat is influenced by hormones like estrogen, giving females their characteristic body shape.

Q. 126. **Why does the superficial fascia act as a distributing layer for blood vessels, lymphatics, and nerves?**

Answer: The superficial fascia acts as a distributing layer for blood vessels, lymphatics, and nerves because of following reason:
- It lies just beneath the skin and serves as a connective tissue layer that supports.
- It separates the skin from the underlying muscles and structures.
- This fascia provides a flexible and cushioning environment that allows these structures to branch out and distribute throughout the body.
- It ensures that
    - Blood vessels,
    - Lymphatics, and
    - Nerves can reach the skin and other superficial tissues, while also providing protection and insulation.

Q. 127. **Why does the superficial fascia act as a cushion at certain sites of the body?**

Answer: The superficial fascia acts as a cushion at certain sites of the body because of following reason:
- It contains a layer of fat that provides padding and absorbs shock.
- This fat helps protect underlying structures, such as
    - Muscles,
    - Bones, and
    - Organs, from external pressure and impact.
- In areas like the buttocks, palms, and soles of the feet, the thicker layer of fat in the superficial fascia offers extra cushioning to support and protect these regions from frequent pressure and stress.

Q. 128. **Why does superficial fascia facilitate movements of the skin?**
Answer: Superficial fascia facilitates movements of the skin because of following reason:
- It provides a flexible medium through which the skin can slide over underlying structures.

Q. 129. **Why is fat more abundant and evenly distributed in females than in males?**
Answer: Fat is more abundant and evenly distributed in females than in males because of following reason:
- It serves as an energy reserve and contributes to reproductive functions.

Q. 130. **Why does superficial fascia conserve body heat?**
Answer: Superficial fascia conserves body heat because of following reason:
- It contains a layer of adipose (fat) tissue.
- This fat acts as an insulator, reducing heat loss from the body by trapping warm air and preventing it from escaping.

Q. 131. **Why are superficial fascia and fat most distinct in the lower part of the anterior abdominal wall?**
Answer: Superficial fascia and fat are most distinct in the lower part of the anterior abdominal wall because of following reason:
- This area is adapted to store more fat. The fat serves as an energy reserve and provides insulation.
- Additionally, the lower abdomen is more prone to fat accumulation due to hormonal and genetic factors.

Q. 132. **Why does fat fill hollow spaces like the axilla and ischiorectal fossa?**
Answer: Fat fills hollow spaces like the axilla and ischiorectal fossa to provide cushioning and support because of following reason:
- It helps
    - Stabilize and protect underlying structures,
    - Absorbs shocks, and
    - Allows for smooth movement of adjacent tissues.

Deep fascia

Q. 133. **Why is the deep fascia described as a tough, inelastic membrane of fibrous tissue?**

Answer: The deep fascia is described as a tough, inelastic membrane of fibrous tissue because of following reason:
- It is composed primarily of dense connective tissue with tightly packed collagen fibers.
- These collagen fibers give the deep fascia its strength and durability, making it resistant to stretching and deformation.
- This inelasticity helps the deep fascia maintain the structural integrity of
  - Muscles,
  - Bones, and
  - Other underlying tissues, providing
    - Support,
    - Protection, and
    - Compartmentalization within the body.

Q. 134. **Why does the deep fascia send septa between groups of muscles in the limbs?**

Answer: The deep fascia sends septa between groups of muscles in the limbs because of following reason:
- To attach with the periosteum of the bone.
- It allows individual muscle groups to contract independently.
- It slides freely over adjacent muscles.

Q. 135. **Why does the deep fascia form 3 layers in the neck?**

Answer: The deep fascia forms three layers in the neck because of following reason:
- To organize and compartmentalize the various structures within the neck, providing support and protection. These layers are:
4. **Investing layer:** this outermost layer surrounds the entire neck, enclosing muscles like the sternocleidomastoid and trapezius, and helping to define the neck's shape.
5. **Pretracheal layer:** this middle layer surrounds the trachea, esophagus, and thyroid gland, providing a protective compartment for these vital structures.
6. **Prevertebral layer:** this innermost layer covers the vertebral column and associated muscles, offering additional support and stability to the spine.

By forming these distinct layers, the deep fascia ensures that the different structures in the neck are securely held in place, allowing for efficient movement and function while protecting them from injury.

Q. 136. **Why does the deep fascia attach to bone wherever it encounters it?**

Answer: The deep fascia attaches to bone wherever it encounters it to provide stability and anchorage for muscles and other structures. This attachment helps
- To transmit the force generated by muscles during movement.
- It ensures that the muscles can effectively exert their action on the bones.
- By anchoring to the bone, the deep fascia also helps to compartmentalize muscles.
- It prevents excessive movement of tissues, maintaining the organization and functional integrity of the musculoskeletal system.

Q. 137. **Why does the deep fascia form retinacula at certain sites?**

Answer: The deep fascia forms retinacula at certain sites
- To hold tendons in place as they pass over joints.
- Retinacula are thickened bands of fascia that prevent the tendons from bowing outward when muscles contract, ensuring that the tendons remain close to the bones.
- This arrangement allows for efficient transmission of force from the muscles to the bones, contributing to precise and controlled movements.
- Retinacula are especially important in areas like the wrist and ankle, where multiple tendons pass over joints and need to be stabilized.

Q. 138. **Why does the deep fascia thicken to form aponeurosis in palms and soles?**

Answer: The deep fascia thickens to form aponeuroses in the palms and soles
- To provide
  - Strength,
  - Stability, and
  - Protection in these areas that experience frequent stress and pressure.
- These thickened sheets of fibrous tissue help distribute the forces exerted on the hands and feet during activities like
  - Gripping,
  - Walking, and
  - Running.
- In the palms, the palmar aponeurosis supports the skin and underlying structures, enhancing grip and preventing slippage.
- In the soles, the plantar aponeurosis helps maintain the arches of the foot, providing support and shock absorption.

Q. 139. **Why does the deep fascia condense to form fibrous sheaths around neurovascular bundles?**
Answer: The deep fascia condenses to form fibrous sheaths around neurovascular bundles of following reason:
- Such as the carotid sheath and axillary sheath, to provide
    - Structural support and
    - Protection while allowing veins to distend.

Q. 140. **Why does the deep fascia split to enclose certain glands?**
Answer: The deep fascia splits to enclose certain glands of following reason:
- Fibrous capsules, such as the parotid gland and submandibular gland, to
    - Protect and
    - Support these structures.

Q. 141. **Why is the deep fascia modified to form interosseous membranes in the forearm and leg?**
Answer: The deep fascia is modified to form interosseous membranes in the forearm and leg of following reason:
- To bind adjacent bones together and
- Maintain their alignment.

Q. 142. **Why does the deep fascia send intermuscular septa in the limbs?**
Answer: The deep fascia sends intermuscular septa in the limbs of following reason:
- To help form compartments for muscles. ,
- It allows groups of muscles to function independently.

Q. 143. **Why does the deep fascia thicken to form fibrous flexor sheaths on the flexor surfaces of fingers and toes?**
Answer: The deep fascia thickens to form fibrous flexor sheaths on the flexor surfaces of fingers and toes of following reason:
- To prevent long flexor tendons from bowing out of position during movement.

Q. 144. **Why are ligaments considered as localized thickened bands of the deep fascia?**
Answer: Ligaments are considered as localized thickened bands of the deep fascia because of following reason:
- They provide additional support and stability to joints,
- They function similarly to the deep fascia in other areas of the body.

Q. 145. **Why does the deep fascia form fascial sheaths around certain muscles, such as the psoas sheath?**

Answer: The deep fascia forms fascial sheaths around certain muscles,
- Such as the psoas sheath, to provide
    - Support,
    - Protection, and
    - Facilitate smooth movement.
- These sheaths encase the muscles, helping to maintain their shape and alignment during contraction and relaxation.
- The fascial sheath also reduces friction between the muscle and surrounding tissues, allowing for efficient movement.
- Additionally, by compartmentalising the muscles, the fascial sheath can help contain the spread of infections or inflammation. It provides an added layer of protection to the body.

Q. 146. **Why is the deep fascia absent at certain sites, such as the face and breast?**

Answer: The deep fascia is absent at certain sites, such as the face and breast,
- To allow for
    - Greater flexibility,
    - Movement, and
    - Accommodation of underlying structures.
- In the face, the absence of deep fascia allows for a wide range of facial expressions by providing the muscles of facial expression the freedom to move the overlying skin directly.
- In the breast, the lack of deep fascia allows
    - The breast tissue to expand and
    - Change shape, which is important for functions like
        - Breastfeeding and
        - Responding to hormonal changes.
- Additionally, the absence of deep fascia in these areas permits a softer and more pliable texture, which is important for the aesthetic and functional characteristics of these regions.

Q. 147. **Why is the deep fascia very sensitive?**

Answer: The deep fascia is very sensitive because
- It contains a network of nerve endings, including those that detect
    - Pain,
    - Pressure, and
    - Stretch.
- This sensitivity allows the deep fascia to respond to

- o Mechanical changes and
- o Potential injuries.
- It plays a role in proprioception, helping the body sense and adjust to changes in muscle tension and movement.
- Additionally, the sensitivity of the deep fascia helps protect underlying structures by alerting the body to potential harm or excessive strain.

Q. 148. Why does the deep fascia facilitate venous and lymphatic drainage?
Answer: The deep fascia facilitates venous and lymphatic drainage because of following reason:
- By providing
  - o Pathways and
  - o Support structures for these systems.

Q. 149. Why does the deep fascia retain long tendons in place?
Answer: The deep fascia retains long tendons in place because of following reason:
- To prevent their bowstringing during muscle action.
- It serves as pulleys to enhance their efficiency.

Q. 150. Why does deep fascia help in venous and lymphatic return from the lower limb?
Answer: Deep fascia helps in venous and lymphatic return from the lower limb by
- Creating a pressure gradient that assists blood and lymph flow.
- It tightly encases muscles, which contract during movement, compressing veins and lymphatic vessels.
- It facilitates the return of blood and lymph toward the heart.

Q. 151. Why is deep fascia important for maintaining the surface contour of the limbs and neck?
Answer: Deep fascia is important for maintaining the surface contour of the limbs and neck because of following reason:
- It keeps underlying structures in position and supports the characteristic appearance of these body parts.

Q. 152. Why are retinacula important in the limbs?
Answer: Retinacula are important in the limbs because
- They act as strong bands of connective tissue that hold tendons in place during movement.
- This prevents the tendons from slipping out of their proper positions, ensuring efficient and controlled movement of the joints and muscles.

Q. 153. **Why does deep fascia form fibroareolar sheaths around muscles, vessels, and nerves?**

Answer: Deep fascia forms fibroareolar sheaths around muscles, vessels, and nerves because of following reason:
- To provide support and protection to these structures within the compartments of the body.

Q. 154. **Why does deep fascia form interosseous membranes in the forearm and leg?**

Answer: Deep fascia forms interosseous membranes in the forearm and leg because of following reason:
- To keep bones at an optimum distance, increase the surface area for muscle attachment, and transmit weight from one bone to another.

Miscellaneous questions

Q. 155. **Why are flexure (joint) lines major markings found in the vicinity of synovial joints?**

Answer: Flexure (joint) lines are major markings found in the vicinity of synovial joints because of following reason:

- They accommodate the skin's movement and folding at these areas of frequent bending.
- These lines help the skin to
    - Flex and
    - Stretch more effectively around the joints.
- It prevents stress and damage to the skin as it moves with the underlying joints and muscles.

Q. 156. **Why does wound healing often involve the coordination of numerous cell types, signalling molecules, and matrix proteins**

Answer: Wound healing often involves the coordination of numerous cell types, signalling molecules, and matrix proteins because of following reason:
- The complex balance of these mediators, rather than their individual action, determines events in wound repair.

Q. 157. **Why is wound contraction an important part of remodelling in wound healing?**

Answer: Wound contraction is an important part of remodelling in wound healing because of following reason:
- Myofibroblasts generated from activated fibroblasts play a key role in pulling normal dermal and adipose tissue.
- They migrate into the wound defect.
- They help to scar formation.

Q. 158. **Why does revascularization of grafts depend on early and direct connection between host and graft vessels?**

Answer: Revascularization of grafts depends on early and direct connection between host and graft vessels because of following reason:
- This connection is crucial for restoring blood supply to the graft.
- The graft needs an adequate blood supply to receive oxygen and nutrients and to remove waste products.
- Early and direct vascular connection helps to ensure the graft survives. It integrates with the surrounding tissue.
- It reduces the risk of graft failure and promoting successful healing.

Q. 159. **Why does the skin contain stem cells in various parts of the hair follicles, basal layer of the interfollicular epidermis, and within sweat glands?**

Answer: The skin contains stem cells in various parts, such as
- Hair follicles,
- The basal layer of the interfollicular epidermis, and
- Within sweat glands, because
- These cells are crucial for
    - Tissue repair and
    - Regeneration.
- When the skin is damage, these stem cells can divide and differentiate into various cell types needed to heal wounds and maintain the skin's integrity.

Q. 160. **Why is the skin regarded as an important organ of the body?**

Answer: The skin is regarded as an important organ of the body because of following reason:
- It performs a large number of essential functions, including
    - Protection,
    - Sensation,
    - Temperature regulation, and
    - Synthesis of vitamin D, making it crucial for overall health and homeostasis.

Q. 161. **Why does the colour of the skin depend on the vascularity of the dermis and the thickness of the keratin in white races?**

Answer: The color of the skin in white races depends on the vascularity of the dermis and the thickness of the keratin because of following reason:
- These factors influence how light is absorbed and reflected by the skin.
- **Vascularity of the dermis**: Blood vessels in the dermis can give the skin a pinkish or reddish hue depending on the amount of blood flow.
    - This effect is more noticeable in people with lighter skin, where the underlying blood vessels are more visible.
- **Thickness of the keratin**: The thickness of the keratin layer in the epidermis can affect how much of this underlying color is visible.
    - Thicker keratin can make the skin appear paler, as it blocks some of the color from the blood vessels.

Together, these factors contribute to the overall color of the skin

Q. 162. **Why does the thickness of the skin vary from about 0.5 to 3 mm?**

Answer: The thickness of the skin varies from about 0.5 to 3 mm because of following reason:
- Different body areas require different levels of protection and flexibility.
- Thicker skin, such as on the palms and soles, provides greater protection and durability,
- Thinner skin in other areas allows for greater sensitivity and flexibility.

Q. 163. **Why does the skin have surface irregularities like tension lines, flexure lines, and papillary ridges?**

Answer: The skin has surface irregularities like tension lines, flexure lines, and papillary ridges because of following reason:
- These features help
    - Accommodate movement,
    - Improve grip, and
    - Enhance the skin's ability to
        - Stretch and

- Return to its original shape.
- Tension lines correspond to underlying fiber patterns.
- , Flexure lines occur at joints, and papillary ridges provide friction ridges for better tactile sensation and grip.

Q. 164. **Why do the epidermis of the skin, hair, nails, cornea of the eye, lens, articular hyaline cartilages, splenic pulp, brain and spinal cord, and bone marrow lack blood capillaries?**

Answer: The epidermis of the skin, hair, nails, cornea of the eye, lens, articular hyaline cartilage, splenic pulp, brain and spinal cord, and bone marrow lack blood capillaries because they are either avascular tissues or specialized regions where direct blood supply could interfere with their function.

7. **Epidermis of the skin, hair, and nails**: These tissues are avascular, meaning they do not have blood vessels.
    - Nutrients and oxygen are supplied through diffusion from the underlying dermis.
    - This arrangement helps protect against injury and infection, as it limits direct access to the bloodstream.
8. **Cornea and lens of the eye**: These structures need to be transparent to allow light to pass through for vision.
    - Blood vessels would obstruct this transparency.
    - They rely on diffusion of nutrients from surrounding fluids, like the aqueous humor.
9. **Articular hyaline cartilage**: This cartilage covers the ends of bones in joints.
    - **It** must be smooth and resilient to reduce friction and absorb shock.
    - Blood vessels would interfere with these mechanical properties.
    - So the cartilage is nourished by synovial fluid in the joint.
10. **Splenic pulp**: The splenic pulp consists mainly of red and white pulp.
    - It filters blood and produce immune responses.
    - The spleen is highly vascularized
    - The specific tissue arrangement avoids direct blood capillaries within the pulp to facilitate its filtering and immune functions.
11. **Brain and spinal cord**: These structures are protected by the blood-brain barrier.
    - **It** regulates the passage of substances from the blood to the nervous tissue.
    - Capillaries in the brain and spinal cord have special properties that maintain this barrier.
    - It reduces the risk of harmful substances entering the nervous system.

12. **Bone marrow**: Bone marrow is highly vascularized overall, but the areas where blood cell production occurs are separated from the capillaries by a specialized structure.
    - This allows for the controlled release of new blood cells into circulation.

In all these cases, the lack of direct blood capillaries is an adaptation to preserve the function and integrity of the tissue or organ.

Q. 165.   **Why the labia minora are termed sex skin?**
Answer: The labia minora are termed "sex skin" because of following reason:
- They are sensitive to hormonal changes and respond to sexual stimulation.
- These inner folds of the vulva are rich in blood vessels and nerve endings, making them highly responsive to sexual arousal.
- During sexual activity, the labia minora can swell and change color due to increased blood flow, which is why they are referred to as "sex skin."

Q. 166.   **Why the face is considered the commonest site of skin cancer?**
Answer: The face is considered the commonest site of skin cancer because of following reason:
- It is frequently exposed to ultraviolet (UV) radiation from the sun.
- The skin on the face is often unprotected, making it more vulnerable to the damaging effects of UV rays.
- It can cause mutations in skin cells and lead to the development of cancer.
- Additionally, the face has a high density of skin cells that are prone to cancer, such as basal and squamous cells, increasing the risk of skin cancer in this area.

Q. 167.   **Why moles are considered the commonest congenital disorder of the skin?**
Answer: Moles are considered the most common congenital disorder of the skin because of following reason:
- They often appear as harmless pigmented spots or growths at birth or develop shortly after.
- They result from an overgrowth of melanocytes,
- Melanocytes are responsible for pigment in the skin.
- While most moles are benign, their prevalence and ease of detection make them a common example of skin disorders that people are born with or acquire early in life.

Q. 168. **Why the mammary gland is considered the largest modified gland of the skin in females?**

Answer: The mammary gland is considered the largest modified gland of the skin in females because of following reason:
- It originates from the skin's sweat glands and undergoes significant development.
- It is large compared to other skin glands due to its role in producing milk, which involves complex structures and extensive tissue growth.
- This functional adaptation makes it notably larger and more specialized than other modified skin glands.

Q. 169. **Why Pacinian corpuscles are considered the largest sensory receptors of the skin?**

Answer: Pacinian corpuscles are considered the largest sensory receptors of the skin because of following reason:
- They detect deep pressure and vibration, located in the deeper layers of the skin.

Q. 170. **Why a lipoma is considered the most common tumor arising from subcutaneous tissue?**

Answer: A lipoma is considered the most common tumor arising from subcutaneous tissue Because of following reason:
- It is a benign growth of fatty tissue that frequently occurs under the skin.

Q. 171. **Why is the Malpighian layer significant in dermatology?**

Answer: The Malpighian layer, or germinative layer of the epidermis, is significant because of following reason:
- It is the site of cell division and the generation of new skin cells.
- It indicates its importance in skin regeneration and repair.

Q. 172. **Why do wounds of the skin heal quickly?**

Answer: Wounds of the skin heal quickly due to because of following reason:
- The skin's ability to regenerate and repair itself.
- The skin has a rich supply of blood vessels that deliver nutrients and oxygen essential for healing.
- Additionally, the skin's cells proliferate rapidly to cover the wound, and various growth factors and immune cells help manage inflammation and prevent infection.

Q. 173. **Why is skin cancer most often associated with the face and neck regions?**

Answer: Skin cancer is most often associated with the face and neck regions because of following reason:

- These areas are usually not covered, making them more exposed to ultraviolet radiation from the sun.

Q. 174. **Why do incisions made parallel to cleavage lines result in less unsightly scars?**

Answer: Incisions made parallel to cleavage lines result in less unsightly scars because of following reason:
- They sever fewer collagen fibers.
- They have decrease tendency of the fibers to retract and resulting in a finer, hairline scar.

8. Tissue

Epithelial Tissue

Q. 1. Why does epithelial tissue have a crucial role in protecting the body?

Answer: Epithelial tissue has a crucial role in protecting the body because of following reason:
- It forms the outer layer of the skin and
- Lines the cavities and surfaces of organs.
- It provides a barrier against
    - Physical damage,
    - Pathogens, and
    - Dehydration, thus maintaining the body's integrity.

Q. 2. Why does the epithelium rest on the basement membrane?

Answer: The epithelium rests on the basement membrane because of following reason:
- The basement membrane provides structural support.
- It anchors the epithelial cells.
- It facilitates nutrient exchange and maintaining tissue integrity.

Q. 3. Why are the cells of the epithelium tightly packed together with little or no intercellular matrix?

Answer: The cells of the epithelium are tightly packed together with little or no intercellular matrix because of following reason:
- This arrangement forms a continuous and effective barrier, protecting underlying tissues from pathogens, toxins, and physical trauma.

Q. 4. Why does epithelium cover body surfaces and line body cavities?

Answer: Epithelium covers body surfaces and lines body cavities because of following reason:
- It serves as a protective layer.
- It prevents infection and fluid loss.
- It facilitates absorption and secretion functions in various organs and systems.

Q. 5. **Why is the high regeneration capacity of epithelial tissue significant?**
Answer: The high regeneration capacity of epithelial tissue is significant because of following reason:
- It ensures rapid repair and replacement of damaged cells.
- It, maintains the integrity and function of the epithelial barrier, which is essential for protection and homeostasis.

Q. 6. **Why does epithelial tissue line tubules such as the gastrointestinal tract and respiratory tract?**
Answer: Epithelial tissue lines tubules such as the gastrointestinal tract and respiratory tract because of following reason:
- It acts as a selective barrier.
- It, facilitates
    - Absorption,
    - Secretion, and
    - Protection against harmful substances and pathogens.

Q. 7. **Why does the epithelium form glands like exocrine and endocrine glands?**
Answer: The epithelium forms glands like exocrine and endocrine glands because of following reason:
- These glands are essential for secreting substances such as hormones and enzymes.
- They regulate various physiological processes and maintain homeostasis.

Q. 8. **Why is simple epithelium composed of a single layer of cells?**
Answer: Simple epithelium is composed of a single layer of cells because of following reason:
- It facilitates
    - Efficient diffusion,
    - Absorption, and
    - Filtration processes, which are essential in areas like blood vessels and alveoli.

Q. 9. Why are simple squamous epithelial cells flattened?
Answer: Simple squamous epithelial cells are flattened because of following reason:
- Their thin structure allows for rapid exchange of gases and nutrients.
- It makes them ideal for lining surfaces involved in diffusion, such as the alveoli of the lungs.

Q. 10. Why does simple columnar epithelium line the gastrointestinal tract?
Answer: Simple columnar epithelium lines the gastrointestinal tract because of following reason:
- Its tall, column-like cells are well-suited for
    - Absorbing nutrients and
    - Secreting digestive enzymes and mucus.
- They are crucial for digestion.

Q. 11. Why does simple ciliated columnar epithelium have cilia on its free surface?
Answer: Simple ciliated columnar epithelium has cilia on its free surface because of following reason:
- The cilia help to move mucus and other substances across the epithelial surface.
- It is particularly important in the respiratory tract and central nervous system.

Q. 12. Why is pseudostratified ciliated columnar epithelium given a stratified appearance?
Answer: Pseudostratified ciliated columnar epithelium is given a stratified appearance because of following reason:
- Its nuclei are positioned at different levels.
- It creates an illusion of multiple layers, which helps in trapping and moving particles out of the respiratory passages.

Q. 13. Why is it termed pseudostratified when the epithelium is not truly stratified?
Answer: It is termed pseudostratified when the epithelium is not truly stratified because of following reason:
- Despite having nuclei at different levels, all cells are in contact with the basement membrane, making it a single layer that appears multi-layered.

Q. 14. **Why does stratified squamous epithelium have squamous cells in its surface layer?**

Answer: Stratified squamous epithelium has squamous cells in its surface layer because of following reason:
- These flattened cells provide a durable and protective barrier against mechanical stress and abrasion.

Q. 15. **Why is stratified squamous nonkeratinized epithelium found in moist areas like the oral cavity and vagina?**

Answer: Stratified squamous nonkeratinized epithelium is found in moist areas like the oral cavity and vagina because of following reason:
- Its non-keratinized cells remain alive and hydrated, which is essential for maintaining the moist environment and protective barrier in these areas.

Q. 16. **Why does stratified squamous keratinized epithelium undergo keratinization?**

Answer: Stratified squamous keratinized epithelium undergoes keratinization because of following reason:
- It needs to provide a tough, impermeable barrier to protect against environmental factors like dryness and pathogens.
- It is crucial for the epidermis of the skin.

Q. 17. **Why is stratified cuboidal epithelium found in ducts of sweat glands and seminiferous tubules?**

Answer: Stratified cuboidal epithelium is found in ducts of sweat glands and seminiferous tubules because of following reason:
- The cube-shaped cells offer
  - Structural support and
  - Protection while allowing the transport of substances through these ducts.

Q. 18. **Why is stratified columnar epithelium present in large ducts of glands?**

Answer: Stratified columnar epithelium is present in large ducts of glands because of following reason:
- Its columnar cells provide a sturdy lining that can withstand the mechanical stress of transporting glandular secretions.

Q. 19. **Why does transitional epithelium exhibit 2 types of transitions in cell shape and number of layers?**

Answer: Transitional epithelium exhibits 2 types of transitions in cell shape and number of layers because of following reason:
- It needs to accommodate the stretching and relaxing of the urinary tract organs, allowing them to expand and contract without losing integrity.

Q. 20. **Why does transitional epithelium have a high number of cell layers when the organ is relaxed?**

Answer: Transitional epithelium has a high number of cell layers when the organ is relaxed because of following reason:
- The additional layers provide structural support and protection, which can then be reduced when the organ is stretched.

Q. 21. **Why transitional epithelium is considered a special variety of stratified epithelium?**

Answer: Transitional epithelium is considered a special variety of stratified epithelium because of following reason:
- Unlike regular stratified epithelium, it can undergo significant changes in shape and layer thickness, adapting to the stretching and relaxing of urinary organs.

Q. 22. **Why does transitional epithelium line organs like the ureter and urinary bladder?**

Answer: Transitional epithelium lines organs like the ureter and urinary bladder because of following reason:
- Its unique ability to stretch and contract is essential for the proper functioning and protection of these organs as they store and transport urine.

Q. 23. **Why do microvilli increase the surface area of the cell membrane?**

Answer: Microvilli increase the surface area of the cell membrane because of following reason:
- This enhances the cell's ability to absorb nutrients and other substances, which is crucial for the functioning of cells lining organs like the small intestine and gallbladder.

Q. 24. **Why are stereocilia considered non-motile despite being long microvilli?**
Answer: Stereocilia are considered non-motile because of following reason:
- They lack the core of actin filaments that provide motility, thus they are primarily involved in absorption and sensory functions rather than movement.

Q. 25. **Why do cilia contain a core of microtubules arranged in a 9+2 pattern?**
Answer: Cilia contain a core of microtubules arranged in a 9+2 pattern because of following reason:
- This specific arrangement is necessary for their motility, enabling them to move substances like mucus in the respiratory tract or ova in the fallopian tubes.

Q. 26. **Why is there always a film of mucus on the free surface of ciliary cells in the respiratory tract?**
Answer: There is always a film of mucus on the free surface of ciliary cells in the respiratory tract because of following reason:
- This mucus traps dust, pathogens, and other particles.
- These are then moved toward the pharynx by the action of the cilia to keep the airways clear.

Q. 27. **Why are glands composed of epithelial cells?**
Answer: Glands are composed of epithelial cells because these cells because of following reason:
- Specialized to produce and secrete fluids that differ in composition from blood or intercellular fluid, which is essential for various physiological processes.

Q. 28. **Why do microvilli have a layer of glycoprotein coating them?**
Answer: Microvilli have a layer of glycoprotein coating them because of following reason:
- This glycocalyx layer helps in protecting the cell surface.
- It facilitates absorption by binding specific molecules.
- It enhances the efficiency of nutrient uptake.

Q. 29. **Why do ciliary cells in the fallopian tubes move the ova towards the uterine cavity?**

Answer: Ciliary cells in the fallopian tubes move the ova towards the uterine cavity because of following reason:
- This movement is essential for the transportation of the ova to the site where fertilization and implantation can occur, ensuring reproductive success.

Q. 30. **Why do goblet cells exist in isolation among nonsecretory cells of the epithelium?**

Answer: Goblet cells exist in isolation among nonsecretory cells of the epithelium because of following reason:
- They provide localized secretion of mucus, which lubricates and protects the lining of organs such as the respiratory tract and intestines.

Q. 31. **Why are exocrine glands termed as glands with ducts?**

Answer: Exocrine glands are termed as glands with ducts because of following reason:
- Their secretions reach the surface epithelium through tubular ducts lined by epithelial cells.
- They allow the secreted substances to be delivered to specific target areas.

Q. 32. **Why do endocrine glands lose their connection with the surface epithelium?**

Answer: Endocrine glands lose their connection with the surface epithelium because of following reason:
- Their secretions, such as hormones, are released directly into the bloodstream.
- It distributes these substances throughout the body to regulate various physiological processes.

Q. 33.   **Why do unicellular glands, like goblet cells, secrete mucus?**
Answer: Unicellular glands, like goblet cells, secrete mucus because of following reason:
- Mucus serves to
    - Lubricate and
    - Protect epithelial surfaces from
        - Mechanical damage,
        - Pathogens, and
        - Dehydration.

Q. 34.   **Why is the mucous lining of the stomach composed of a coherent sheet of epithelial cells?**
Answer: The mucous lining of the stomach is composed of a coherent sheet of epithelial cells because of following reason:
- This continuous layer provides a robust barrier.
- It produces consistent secretion of mucus to protect the stomach lining from acidic gastric juices and mechanical damage.

Q. 35.   **Why do exocrine gland secretions reach the surface through ducts?**
Answer: Exocrine gland secretions reach the surface through ducts because of following reason:
- The ducts provide a direct pathway for the secretion to be transported to specific locations where it performs its intended function, such as lubricating or protecting epithelial surfaces.

Q. 36.   **Why are endocrine glands also known as ductless glands?**
Answer: Endocrine glands are known as ductless glands because of following reason:
- They release their secretions directly into the bloodstream rather than through ducts.
- They enable the hormones to be quickly transported to distant target organs and tissues.

Connective Tissue

Q. 37. **Why does connective tissue play a vital role in supporting and connecting other tissues?**

Answer: Connective tissue plays a vital role in supporting and connecting other tissues because of following reason:
- It provides
    - Structural and
    - Metabolic support.
- It, forms the framework that holds tissues and organs together, thereby ensuring stability and function of the body's systems.

Q. 38. **Why is ground substance important in connective tissue?**

Answer: Ground substance is important in connective tissue because of following reason:
- It fills the space between cells and fibers.
- It provides Ito a medium for nutrient and waste exchange, and supporting tissue resilience and flexibility.

Q. 39. **Why are collagen fibers essential in connective tissue?**

Answer: Collagen fibers are essential in connective tissue because of following reason:
- They provide tensile strength and support, making them crucial for the structural integrity of tissues like tendons, ligaments, and bones.

Q. 40. **Why do elastic fibers provide elasticity to tissues?**

Answer: Elastic fibers provide elasticity to tissues because of following reason:
- They can stretch and recoil, which is vital for the function of tissues that undergo frequent stretching, such as the skin, lungs, and blood vessels.

Q. 41. **Why do reticular fibers form delicate networks?**

Answer: Reticular fibers form delicate networks because of following reason:
- Their fine, branching structure supports the framework of soft organs like the spleen, lymph nodes, and bone marrow, facilitating cellular organization and function.

Q. 42. **Why are fibroblasts important in wound healing?**
Answer: Fibroblasts are important in wound healing because of following reason:
- They actively produce collagen and other matrix components.
- These help in tissue repair and the formation of new extracellular matrix, thus aiding in the healing process.

Q. 43. **Why are macrophages crucial in connective tissue?**
Answer: Macrophages are crucial in connective tissue because of following reason:
- They perform phagocytic functions.
- They, engulf and digesting pathogens, dead cells, and debris.
- They are essential for maintaining tissue health and immune defense.

Q. 44. **Why do mast cells play a role in hypersensitivity reactions?**
Answer: Mast cells play a role in hypersensitivity reactions because of following reason:
- They release histamine and other mediators upon activation.
- They cause
    - Vasodilation,
    - Increased vascular permeability, and
    - Smooth muscle contraction.
- These features are characteristic of allergic responses.

Q. 45. **Why do adipocytes store lipids?**
Answer: Adipocytes store lipids because of following reason:
- They serve as energy reserves.
- They, provide fuel for the body, and play a role in cushioning and insulating organs.

Q. 46. **Why are melanocytes important in protecting tissues?**
Answer: Melanocytes are important in protecting tissues because of following reason:
- They produce melanin, a pigment that
    - Absorbs and dissipates ultraviolet radiation,
    - Preventing DNA damage in skin cells.

Q. 47. **Why is reticular connective tissue significant in certain organs?**
Answer: Reticular connective tissue is significant in certain organs because of following reason:
- Its network of reticular fibers provides a supportive framework.
- This helps to maintain the structure and function of organs like
    - The spleen,
    - Lymph nodes, and
    - Bone marrow.

Q. 48. **Why is connective tissue considered to have a versatile function in the body?**
Answer: Connective tissue is considered versatile because of following reason:
- It provides structural support
- It aids in repair, defense.
- It serves as a medium for
    - The transport of nutrients and
    - Waste through its loose texture and vascular pathways.

Q. 49. **Why are collagen diseases characterized by fibrinoid necrosis?**
Answer: Collagen diseases are characterized by fibrinoid necrosis because of following reason:
- The immune-mediated inflammation targets the connective tissue.
- It leads to the destruction and necrosis of collagen fibers.

Q. 50. **Why does scleroderma lead to thickness and firmness of the skin?**
Answer: Scleroderma leads to thickness and firmness of the skin because of following reason:
- There is excessive deposition of fibrous tissue in the dermis.
- It stiffens and hardens the affected areas.

Q. 51. **Why do neuropathic joints lose stability?**
Answer: Neuropathic joints lose stability because of following reason:
- The nerve damage associated with conditions like tabes dorsalis affects the normal feedback mechanisms.
- Nerves control joint movement and stability, leading to abnormal joint function.

Q. 52.   **Why collagen is considered the most abundant protein in the body?**
Answer: Collagen is considered the most abundant protein in the body because of following reason:
- it is a major component of connective tissues, including
    - Skin,
    - Tendons,
    - Ligaments,
    - Cartilage, and
    - Bones.
- It provides
    - Structural support,
    - Strength, and
    - Elasticity to these tissues.
- Collagen makes up about 25-30% of the total protein content in the human body
- It is essential for maintaining the structure and function of various organs and tissues.

Q. 53.   **Why a lipoma is considered the most common tumor arising from subcutaneous tissue?**
Answer: A lipoma is considered the most common tumor arising from subcutaneous tissue because of following reason:
- It is a benign growth of fat cells (adipocytes) that occurs just beneath the skin.
- Lipomas are the most frequently encountered soft tissue tumors in clinical practice due to the **abundance of adipose tissue in** the body.
- They are typically slow-growing, painless, and often found in areas like the neck, shoulders, back, and arms, making them the most common type of tumor in subcutaneous tissue.

Muscle Tissue

Q. 54. **Why is muscle tissue made up of specialized contractile cells?**
Answer: Muscle tissue is made up of specialized contractile cells because of following reason:
- These cells contain proteins like actin and myosin, which enable the cells to contract and generate force.
- This ability to contract is essential
    - For movement,
    - Maintaining posture, and
    - various vital functions such as
        - Pumping blood and
        - Facilitating digestion.

Q. 55. **Why are there 3 types of muscle tissue?**
Answer: There are three types of muscle tissue because of following reason:
- Each type serves a different function:
    - Skeletal muscle for voluntary movements,
    - Smooth muscle for involuntary actions in organs, and
    - Cardiac muscle for heart contractions.

Q. 56. **Why are muscle fibers crucial for muscle tissue?**
Answer: Muscle fibers are crucial for muscle tissue because of following reason:
- They possess the ability to contract.
- This is essential for generating the force needed for movement and stability in the body.

Q. 57. **Why is the study of muscle tissue divided into skeletal, smooth, and cardiac muscles?**
Answer: The study of muscle tissue is divided into skeletal, smooth, and cardiac muscles because of following reason:
- Each type has distinct structural and functional characteristics that are vital for different physiological roles in the body.

Q. 58.   **Why are muscle fibers referred to as contractile cells?**
Answer: Muscle fibers are referred to as contractile cells because of following reason:
- They have the unique ability to shorten and generate force, which is essential for muscle contraction and movement.

Q. 59.   **Why does tissue regeneration occur by replication of original cells?**
Answer: Tissue regeneration occurs by replication of original cells because of following reason:
- To maintain the function and integrity of tissues.
- The body needs to restore the specific structure and function of the damaged tissue.
- Replicating the original cells ensures that the regenerated tissue closely matches the original in both form and function.

Nervous Tissue

Q. 60.   **Why neurons are considered excitable cells?**
Answer: Neurons are considered excitable cells because of following reason:
- They can initiate, receive, conduct, and transmit electrical signals.
- These are essential for communication within the nervous system.

Q. 61.   **Why do neurons and neuroglia make up nervous tissue?**
Answer: Neurons and neuroglia make up nervous tissue because of following reason:
- Neurons are responsible for transmitting information.
- The neuroglia provide the necessary
    - Structural and
    - Functional support to maintain neuronal health and function.

Q. 62.   **Why do neuroglia provide support to neurons?**
Answer: Neuroglia provide support to neurons because of following reason:
- They are non-excitable cells that help
    - Maintain the homeostasis,
    - Protect the nervous system from pathogens, and
    - Ensure the proper functioning of neural networks.

Q. 63. **Why is the function of neurons significant in nervous tissue?**
Answer: The function of neurons is significant in nervous tissue because of following reason:
- They are the primary cells responsible for transmitting information throughout the body,
    - Enabling sensory perception,
    - Motor control, and
    - Cognitive processes.

Q. 64. **Why do neuroglia play a vital role in the nervous system?**
Answer: Neuroglia play a vital role in the nervous system because of following reason:
- They support and protect neurons, regulate the extracellular environment, and assist in the repair and development of nervous tissue.

Regeneration and Repair

Q. 65. **Why does the rate of regeneration depend on the normal rate of physiological turnover of particular types of cells?**
Answer: The rate of regeneration depends on the normal rate of physiological turnover of particular types of cells because of following reason:
- Cells with a higher turnover rate can regenerate faster, ensuring rapid healing and replacement.

Q. 66. **Why do labile cells regenerate very fast?**
Answer: Labile cells regenerate very fast because of following reason:
- Their replication is a continuous process.
- It allows quick replacement of cells in tissues that frequently experience wear and tear, such as
    - The epithelium of the skin and
    - Mucous membranes.

Q. 67.   **Why are stable cells capable of replication but do so infrequently?**
Answer: Stable cells are capable of replication but do so infrequently because of following reason:
- They do not regularly undergo turnover; however, they can proliferate when needed, such as in
    o Response to injury or
    o Increased demand.

Q. 68.   **Why permanent cells are incapable of replicating after normal growth is complete?**
Answer: Permanent cells are incapable of replicating after normal growth is complete because of following reason:
- They have exited the cell cycle.
- They have entered a phase where they no longer divide.
- This is due to their highly specialized functions, which limit their ability to re-enter the cycle of growth and division.
- They lose their ability to divide, making them unable to regenerate once they reach maturity, as seen in nerve cells and cardiac muscle cells.

Q. 69.   **Why is the division into labile, stable, and permanent cells significant for understanding tissue regeneration?**
Answer: The division into labile, stable, and permanent cells is significant for understanding tissue regeneration because of following reason:
- The division into labile, stable, and permanent cells is significant for understanding tissue regeneration because it helps explain how different tissues respond to injury.
- Labile cells continuously divide and can easily regenerate,
- Stable cells divide only when needed, and
- Permanent cells do not divide at all.
- This classification determines the regenerative capacity of different tissues and informs treatment strategies for tissue repair.

Q. 70. **Why are the cells of the epithelium, bone marrow, blood, spleen, and lymphoid tissue considered labile?**

Answer: The cells of the epithelium, bone marrow, blood, spleen, and lymphoid tissue are considered labile because of following reason:
- They continuously replicate.
- They help rapid regeneration to maintain
    - Tissue function and
    - Respond to damage.

Q. 71. **Why do liver, kidney, and pancreatic cells, along with fibroblasts, smooth muscle cells, and bone cells, fall into the category of stable cells?**

Answer: Liver, kidney, and pancreatic cells, along with fibroblasts, smooth muscle cells, and bone cells, fall into the category of stable cells because of following reason:
- They replicate occasionally, allowing for regeneration in response to injury or increased functional demand.

Q. 72. **Why are nerve cells, skeletal muscle cells, and cardiac muscle cells categorized as permanent cells?**

Answer: Nerve cells, skeletal muscle cells, and cardiac muscle cells are categorized as permanent cells because of following reason:
- They do not have the ability to replicate after the normal growth phase, limiting their regenerative capacity.

Q. 73. **Why is understanding the regenerative capacity of different cell types important for medical treatments?**

Answer: Understanding the regenerative capacity of different cell types is important for medical treatments because of following reason:
- It guides strategies for healing based on tissue regenerative potential.
- It aids in tailoring tissue engineering approaches to specific tissues.

Miscellaneous questions

Q. 74. **Why are tissues considered collections of cells performing a similar function?**

Answer: Tissues are considered collections of cells performing a similar function because of following reason:
- They are groups of cells that work together to carry out specific activities or roles within the body.
- Each tissue type is made up of cells that have similar structures and work in unison to perform a common function, such as
    - Protection,
    - Support,
    - Movement, or
    - Communication.

Q. 75. **Why does the term 'tissue' include both collections of cells and intercellular substance?**

Answer: The term 'tissue' includes both collections of cells and intercellular substance because of following reason:
- The intercellular substance provides the necessary support and environment for the cells to function effectively, indicating a collaborative structure for optimal performance.

Q. 76. **Why are epithelial and connective tissues discussed separately from muscle and nervous tissues in the chapter?**

Answer: Epithelial and connective tissues are discussed separately from muscle and nervous tissues because of following reason:
- They have different
    - Structures,
    - Functions, and
    - Roles in the body.
- Epithelial and connective tissues primarily provide
    - Support,
    - Protection, and
    - Connection between different parts of the body, while muscle tissues are responsible for movement, and nervous tissues are involved in communication and control of body functions.

- o The distinct roles and characteristics of these tissue types warrant separate discussions in the chapter.

Q. 77. Why is it important to differentiate between the 4 basic types of tissues in the body?

Answer: It is important to differentiate between the 4 basic types of tissues in the body because of following reason:
- Each type plays a unique role in maintaining the body'
    - o Structure and
    - o Function, hence a clear understanding is essential for studying human anatomy and physiology comprehensively.

Q. 78. Why is simple cuboidal epithelium found in the thyroid follicles and ovary?

Answer: Simple cuboidal epithelium is found in the thyroid follicles and ovary because of following reason:
- These cube-shaped cells provide sufficient volume for the secretion and absorption of substances.
- These are vital functions in these glands.

Q. 79. Why the surface are cells of transitional epithelium large and rounded when the organ is relaxed?

Answer: The surface cells of transitional epithelium are large and rounded when the organ is relaxed because of following reason:
- This shape allows them to stretch and flatten when the organ becomes distended, providing flexibility and maintaining a barrier.

Q. 80. Why do glands produce secretion?

Answer: Glands produce secretion because of following reason:
- Their specialized epithelial cells are adapted to synthesize
- They release substances necessary for various bodily functions, such as
    - o Digestion,
    - o Lubrication, and
    - o Hormone regulation.

Q. 81. **Why are multicellular glands derived from the epithelial lining through proliferation and evagination?**

Answer: Multicellular glands are derived from the epithelial lining through proliferation and evagination because of following reason:
- This process allows the formation of complex glandular structures.
- These structures can produce and secrete larger quantities of substances into ducts or directly into the blood stream.

Q. 82. **Why is connective tissue important for the body's highly organized structures?**

Answer: Connective tissue is important for the body's highly organized structures because of following reason:
- It provides a supporting matrix that acts as packing material.
- It ensures that highly organized structures remain stable and functional.

Q. 83. **Why does the extracellular component of connective tissue serve mechanical functions of support and protection?**

Answer: The extracellular component serves these functions because of following reason:
- It is made up of fibers and ground substance.
- It provides structural integrity and resistance against mechanical stresses and strains.

Q. 84. **Why are sprains visible on X-ray films as normal bones?**

Answer: Sprains are visible on X-ray films as normal bones because of following reason:
- X-rays primarily show bones. It does not show soft tissues like ligaments.
- A sprain involves damage to ligaments. Ligaments are soft tissues that connect bones at a joint.
- Since X-rays don't effectively capture soft tissue details, the bones appear normal even if there's a ligament injury.

Q. 85. **Why loose connective tissue is considered the most widely distributed connective tissue in the body?**

Answer: Loose connective tissue is considered the most widely distributed connective tissue because
- It supports and fills spaces between organs, tissues, and other structures throughout the body.
- It provides a flexible, supportive framework.
- It serves as a cushioning material.
- It helps to hold organs and tissues in place.
- Its widespread presence is essential for maintaining the integrity and function of various body parts.

Q. 86. **Why fibroblasts are considered the most abundant connective tissue cells?**

Answer: Fibroblasts are considered the most abundant connective tissue cells because of following reason:
- They are responsible for producing and maintaining the extracellular matrix.
- It includes collagen, elastin, and other fibers that provide structure and support to tissues.
- They are found in almost all types of connective tissue, making them crucial for
    - Tissue repair,
    - Wound healing, and
    - Overall tissue maintenance.
- Their abundance indicates their essential role in maintaining the structural integrity of connective tissues throughout the body.

Q. 87. **Why enamel is considered the hardest tissue in the body?**

Answer: Enamel is considered the hardest tissue in the body because of following reason:
- It contains a high concentration of minerals, primarily hydroxyapatite. It is a crystalline form of calcium phosphate.
- This mineralization makes enamel extremely strong and resilient.
- It protects the underlying dentin and pulp of teeth from
    - Mechanical forces, such as chewing, and
    - From chemical erosion.
- Its hardness is essential for its role in the body's ability to process food.

9. Endocrine system

Gland-Specific Questions:

1. Why do endocrine glands exist as separate distinct organs like the pituitary, thyroid, and parathyroid glands?

Answer: Endocrine glands exist as separate distinct organs like the pituitary, thyroid, and parathyroid glands because of following reason:

- These organs need to produce and release specific hormones directly into the bloodstream to regulate various bodily functions systematically.

2. Why are there scattered masses of endocrine cells within exocrine glands such as the islets of Langerhans within the pancreas?

Answer: There are scattered masses of endocrine cells within exocrine glands such as the islets of Langerhans within the pancreas because of following reason:

- These endocrine cells need to produce hormones like insulin and glucagon to regulate blood sugar levels.
- The exocrine portion of the pancreas performs digestive functions.

3. Why is it significant that neuroendocrine cells are found in locations like the lining epithelium of the duodenum?

Answer: It is significant that neuroendocrine cells are found in locations like the lining epithelium of the duodenum because of following reason:

- They release hormones that regulate digestive processes and coordinate with the nervous system to ensure proper digestion and nutrient absorption.

4. Why endocrine glands are considered ductless?

Answer: Endocrine glands are considered ductless because of following reason:

- They release their hormones directly into the bloodstream rather than through ducts, allowing for rapid and widespread distribution of hormonal signals throughout the body.

5. Why is the pituitary gland located in the sella turcica?

Answer: The pituitary gland is located in the sella turcica because of following reason:

- This bony fossa provides protection and support for the gland.
- It is closely connected to the hypothalamus for effective endocrine regulation.

6. Why does the parathyroid hormone (PTH) play a crucial role in calcium homeostasis?

Answer: Parathyroid hormone (PTH) plays a crucial role in calcium homeostasis because of following reason:

- It regulates the levels of calcium in the blood by increasing calcium release from bones.
- It enhances calcium absorption in the intestines, and reduces calcium loss in the urine.

7. Why are the suprarenal glands also known as adrenal glands?

Answer: The suprarenal glands are also known as adrenal glands because of following reason:

- They are located on top of the kidneys (renal) and their name "adrenal" literally means "near the kidneys," reflecting their anatomical position.

8. Why does the thymus gland secrete thymosin?

Answer: The thymus gland secretes thymosin because of following reason:

- This hormone is essential for the development and maturation of T lymphocytes, which are critical for the immune system's ability to fight off infections and diseases.

9. Why do the islets of Langerhans contain alpha and beta cells?

Answer: The islets of Langerhans contain alpha and beta cells because of following reason:

- To regulate blood sugar levels through the production of glucagon and insulin, respectively.

10. Why does the pancreas have both exocrine and endocrine functions?
Answer: The pancreas has both exocrine and endocrine functions because of following reason:
- To perform digestion-related activities through the production of digestive enzymes.
- It regulates blood sugar levels through the secretion of hormones like insulin and glucagon.

11. Why are Leydig cells significant in the testes?
Answer: Leydig cells are significant in the testes because of following reason:
- They produce testosterone, which is crucial for the development of male secondary sexual characteristics, maintenance of sperm production, and regulation of GnRH production from the hypothalamus.

12. Why is the corpus luteum important after ovulation?
Answer: The corpus luteum is important after ovulation because of following reason:
- It acts as an endocrine gland, secreting progesterone to maintain the pregnancy until the placenta forms and takes over its function.

13. Why do the juxtaglomerular cells of the kidney produce renin?
Answer: The juxtaglomerular cells of the kidney produce renin because of following reason:
- To regulate blood pressure and fluid balance in the body by activating the renin-angiotensin-aldosterone system.

Hormone-Specific Questions:

14. Why do hormones/chemical messengers need to be classified into different types like proteins, steroids, small peptides, and amino acid derivatives?
Answer: Hormones/chemical messengers need to be classified into different types like proteins, steroids, small peptides, and amino acid derivatives because of following reason:
- Each type has unique properties and mechanisms of action that affect how they interact with target cells and tissues.

15. Why is it crucial for the secretion of endocrine glands to be known as hormones or chemical messengers?

Answer: It is crucial for the secretion of endocrine glands to be known as hormones or chemical messengers because of following reason:
- This terminology accurately reflects their role in transmitting signals that regulate physiological processes and maintain homeostasis.

16. Why is the understanding of factors regulating the secretion of each hormone vital for clinicians?

Answer: Understanding factors regulating the secretion of each hormone is vital for clinicians because of following reason:
- It helps them diagnose endocrine disorders and develop effective treatment plans based on how various stimuli affect hormone production and release.

17. Why does the failure of ADH secretion produce diabetes insipidus?

Answer: The failure of ADH secretion produces diabetes insipidus because of following reason:
- Without ADH, the kidneys cannot properly reabsorb water, leading to excessive urine production and severe thirst as the body tries to compensate for the lost fluids.

18. Why is the secretion of thyroid hormones essential for psychosomatic growth and maintaining basal metabolic rate (BMR)?

Answer: The secretion of thyroid hormones is essential for psychosomatic growth and maintaining basal metabolic rate (BMR) because of following reason:
- These hormones stimulate metabolism, promote normal growth and development, and ensure that the body's cells have the energy needed for their functions.

19. Why do adrenal androgens have a minor importance in males but a significant role in females?

Answer: Adrenal androgens have a minor importance in males because of following reason:
- The primary source of androgens in males is the testes, whereas in females, adrenal androgens contribute to the development of secondary sexual characteristics such as pubic and axillary hair.

20. Why does the secretion of melatonin by the pineal gland inhibit the development of reproductive organs before puberty?

Answer: The secretion of melatonin by the pineal gland inhibits the development of reproductive organs before puberty because of following reason:
- Melatonin suppresses the release of gonadotropin-releasing hormone (GnRH), delaying the onset of puberty until the appropriate time.

21. Why is the hormone progesterone necessary for pregnancy?

Answer: The hormone progesterone is necessary for pregnancy because of following reason:
- It prepares and maintains the endometrium to support the implantation and growth of the fertilized ovum.

22. Why does gastrin act on the fundic glands of the stomach?

Answer: Gastrin acts on the fundic glands of the stomach because of following reason:
- To stimulate the secretion of hydrochloric acid (HCl), which is crucial for the digestion of food and killing of pathogens.

23. Why does secretin affect the pancreas?

Answer: Secretin affects the pancreas because of following reason:
- It stimulates the secretion of pancreatic juice, which contains bicarbonate to neutralize stomach acid and digestive enzymes to aid in digestion.

24. Why is the regulation of acid secretion by enterogastrone important?

Answer: The regulation of acid secretion by enterogastrone is important because of following reason:
- It helps prevent excessive acidity in the stomach, which can lead to ulcers and other gastrointestinal issues.

Structural/ functional classification:

25. Why do chromophils possess secretory granules?

Answer: Chromophils possess secretory granules because of following reason:
- These granules contain the hormones that the cells release into the bloodstream, allowing for the regulation of various physiological processes.

26. Why are basophils classified into thyrotrophs and gonadotrophs based on their function?

Answer: Basophils are classified into thyrotrophs and gonadotrophs based on their function because of following reason:
- Thyrotrophs secrete thyroid-stimulating hormone (TSH) to regulate the thyroid gland.
- Gonadotrophs secrete hormones like FSH and LH to regulate the reproductive organs.

27. Why are enteroendocrine cells found in the epithelial layer of the stomach and small intestine?

Answer: Enteroendocrine cells are found in the epithelial layer of the stomach and small intestine because of following reason:
- They secrete hormones that regulate various aspects of digestion and gut motility.

Miscellaneous

28. Why do the important endocrine glands include the pituitary gland, thymus gland?

Answer: The important endocrine glands include the pituitary gland, thyroid gland, parathyroid glands, suprarenal glands, pineal gland, and thymus gland because of following reason:
- These glands produce key hormones that regulate essential bodily functions such as growth, metabolism, stress response, and immune function.

10. Genetics and radiological anatomy

Genetics

Q. 1.   Why is it important to study genetics in the context of inherited diseases?

Answer: Studying genetics in the context of inherited diseases because of following reason:
- Helps understand how genetic mutations and variations contribute to disease susceptibility and manifestation.

Q. 2.   Why do autosomal dominant diseases require only one copy of the defective gene to manifest?

Answer: Autosomal dominant diseases require only one copy of the defective gene to manifest because of following reason:
- Require only one copy of the defective gene to manifest because the presence of one copy is sufficient to cause the disease phenotype.

Q. 3.   Why cystic fibrosis is considered an autosomal recessive disease?

Answer: Cystic fibrosis is considered an autosomal recessive disease because of following reason:
- It requires two copies of the defective gene (one from each parent) for the disease to be expressed.

Q. 4.   Why are X-linked recessive diseases more commonly observed in males than females?

Answer: X-linked recessive diseases are more commonly observed in males than females because of following reason:
- Males have only one X chromosome, so if it carries a defective gene, they will express the disease phenotype.

Q. 5.   Why is Huntington's disease characterized by a progressive loss of mental activity?

Answer: Huntington's disease is characterized by a progressive loss of mental activity because of following reason:
- It causes degeneration of nerve cells in certain parts of the brain, leading to cognitive decline.

Q. 6. **Why are Klinefelter's syndrome individuals phenotypically male despite having an extra X chromosome?**

Answer: Klinefelter's syndrome individuals are phenotypically male because they have a Y chromosome because of following reason:
- Which determines maleness, and two X chromosomes, which causes mild feminization traits but does not override the male phenotype.

Q. 7. **Why does Turner's syndrome result in short stature and webbing of the neck? AI**

Answer: Turner's syndrome results in short stature and webbing of the neck because of following reason:
- The absence of one X chromosome, which leads to abnormalities in growth and development.

Q. 8. **Why are Duchenne muscular dystrophy patients prone to progressive muscle weakness?**

Answer: Duchenne muscular dystrophy patients are prone to progressive muscle weakness because of following reason:
- The disease causes a lack of dystrophin, a protein necessary for muscle integrity, leading to muscle degeneration.

Q. 9. **Why color blindness is considered an X-linked recessive disorder?**

Answer: Color blindness is considered an X-linked recessive disorder because of following reason:
- The genes responsible for color vision are located on the X chromosome, and a defective copy of the gene on the X chromosome can result in color blindness.

Q. 10. **Why are there no Y-linked diseases transmitted from father to son?**

Answer: There are no Y-linked diseases transmitted from father to son because of following reason:
- The Y chromosome is small and carries relatively few genes.
  Most of the genes are involved in male sex determination and spermatogenesis, rather than general bodily functions.

Radiological anatomy

Q. 11. **Why were x-rays named as "x-rays" at the time of their discovery?**
Answer: X-rays were named "x-rays" because of following reason:
- Wilhelm Conrad Roentgen in 1895 discovered X rays. Nothing was known about their nature. The term "x" stands for unknown, hence they were called x-rays.

Q. 12. **Why do x-rays have the ability to penetrate materials that visible light cannot?**
Answer: X-rays have a much shorter wavelength compared to visible light because of following reason:
- It allows to penetrate materials that absorb or reflect visible light. This characteristic makes x-rays useful for medical imaging.

Q. 13. **Why is the absorption of x-rays greater in dense tissues like bones compared to less dense tissues like soft tissues?**
Answer: X-rays are absorbed more in dense tissues like bones because of following reason:
- These tissues have a higher atomic weight and density.
- This results in less penetration and greater opacity on a radiograph.

Q. 14. **Why does bone appear white (radiopaque) on a radiograph?**
Answer: Bone appears white (radiopaque) on a radiograph because of following reason:
- It absorbs more x-rays compared to surrounding tissues.
- It results in less exposure of the film and a lighter appearance.

Q. 15. **Why are air-filled spaces like the trachea and lungs seen as dark (radiolucent) on a radiograph?**
Answer: Air-filled spaces like the trachea and lungs appear dark (radiolucent) on a radiograph because of following reason:
- They absorb fewer x-rays.
- They allow more exposure of the film and a darker appearance.

Q. 16. **Why do x-rays affect photographic film in a manner similar to visible light waves?**
Answer: X-rays affect photographic film similarly to visible light waves because of following reason:
- Both types of radiation can sensitively affect the silver bromide crystals in the film.
- It produces a visible image after development.

Q. 17. **Why are x-rays used in fluoroscopy to observe movements of internal organs like the lungs and stomach?**
Answer: X-rays are used in fluoroscopy because of following reason:
- When x-rays strike certain substances, they cause them to fluoresce.
- They allow the observation of real-time movements of organs on a fluorescent screen.

Q. 18. **Why are x-rays used in radiotherapy to target and destroy cancer cells?**
Answer: X-rays are used in radiotherapy because of following reason:
- They can destroy abnormal cells, such as cancer cells.
- Cancer cells have higher radio sensitivity than normal cells.

Q. 19. **Why are rapidly growing cells like cancer cells more sensitive to radiation than normal cells?**
Answer: Rapidly growing cells like cancer cells are more sensitive to radiation because of following reason:
- Cancer cells are in a state of active division.
- The DNA of the cell is more vulnerable to the damaging effects of radiation.

Q. 20. **Why are lymphocytes and leucocytes among the most radiosensitive cells in the human body?**
Answer: Lymphocytes and leucocytes are among the most radiosensitive cells because of following reason:
- They are actively dividing and have a high metabolic rate.
- This makes them vulnerable to the effects of ionizing radiation.

Q. 21. **Why are ultrasonic waves used in ultrasonography?**
Answer: Ultrasonic waves are used in ultrasonography because of following reason:
- Their high frequency cannot be heard by the human ear, hence the name ultrasonic waves.

Q. 22. **Why is ultrasound very useful in assessing the nature of masses in the abdomen and soft tissues?**
Answer: Ultrasound is very useful in assessing the nature of masses in the abdomen and soft tissues because of following reason:
- It can differentiate between
    - Solid and
    - Fluid-filled masses.

Q. 23. **Why are gas-filled structures such as the lungs and bowel very difficult to visualize in ultrasound?**
Answer: Gas-filled structures such as the lungs and bowel are very difficult to visualize in ultrasound because of following reason:
- Gas and bone are not suitable for ultrasonography.

Q. 24. **Why is ultrasound now the primary mode of investigating suspected gall-bladder disease?**
Answer: Ultrasound is now the primary mode of investigating suspected gall-bladder disease because of following reason:
- Ultrasonologists simultaneously look at the
    - Liver,
    - Kidneys, and
    - Pancreas.

Q. 25. **Why MRI is considered superior to CT in providing good soft tissue contrast?**
Answer: MRI is considered superior to CT in providing good soft tissue contrast because of following reason:
- It uses strong magnets and radiofrequencies to generate images, rather than x-rays.

Q. 26. Why is MRI the first investigation of choice to detect tumors in the brain and spinal cord?

Answer: MRI is the first investigation of choice to detect tumors in the brain and spinal cord because of following reason:
- It provides detailed images of soft tissues without the use of ionizing radiation.

Q. 27. Why the MRI images are called pictorial representations of the spatial distribution of mobile protons of hydrogen ions?

Answer: The MRI images are called pictorial representations of the spatial distribution of mobile protons of hydrogen ions because of following reason:
- These protons behave like tiny magnets and emit radiofrequencies that are detected by sensitive detectors.

Q. 28. Why is a PET scan used to determine metabolic activity in organs?

Answer: A PET scan is used to determine metabolic activity in organs because of following reason:
- It tracks the movements and concentration of a radioactive tracer injected into the blood.

Q. 29. Why does a PET scan combine computed tomography and nuclear scanning?

Answer: A PET scan combines computed tomography and nuclear scanning because of following reason:
- It reveals metabolic and functional changes at the cellular level in an organ.

Q. 30. Why is a PET scan able to detect metabolic and functional changes early?

Answer: A PET scan is able to detect metabolic and functional changes early because of following reason:
- It detects these changes before structural changes occur in the organ, unlike CT scan or MRI.

Q. 31. **Why do the images on screen or photographic films display shades of grey?**

Answer: The images on screen or photographic films display shades of grey because of following reason:
- They are composed of different densities of tissues ranging from white to black.

Q. 32. **Why do radiologists use different terminologies to describe shades of brightness and darkness in new imaging modalities?**

Answer: Radiologists use different terminologies to describe shades of brightness and darkness in new imaging modalities because of following reason:
- These modalities can distinguish more than the four densities seen in plain radiographs.

Q. 33. **Why are bone, soft tissues, fat, and air represented by different shades in plain radiographs?**

Answer: Bone, soft tissues, fat, and air are represented by different shades in plain radiographs because of following reason:
- They have different densities that reflect X-rays differently.

Q. 34. **Why X-rays are considered a valuable diagnostic tool in medicine?**

Answer: X-rays are considered a valuable diagnostic tool in medicine because of following reason:
- They can penetrate different tissues of the body to varying extents.
- They, allow detailed imaging of internal structures and aid in the detection of early-stage diseases.

Q. 35. **Why must adequate protective measures be taken against repeated exposures to X-rays?**

Answer: Adequate protective measures must be taken against repeated exposures to X-rays because of following reason:
- Repeated exposure can cause harmful biological effects such as burns, tumors, and mutations, posing significant health risks.

Q. 36. **Why are certain structures in X-ray images described as radiolucent and others as radiopaque?**

Answer: Certain structures in X-ray images are described as radiolucent and others as radiopaque because of following reason:
- Radiolucent structures, such as
  - Air and
  - Fat, allow X-rays to pass through easily, producing black shadows,
- Radiopaque structures, like
  - Bones and
  - Teeth, absorb X-rays and produce white shadows.

Q. 37. **Why does the wavelength of X-rays contribute to their penetrating power?**

Answer: The wavelength of X-rays contributes to their penetrating power because
- X-rays have a much shorter wavelength compared to visible light.
- It enables them to penetrate various materials to different extents depending on their density.

Q. 38. **Why does the property of X-rays causing certain metallic salts to fluoresce have practical applications?**

Answer: The property of X-rays causing certain metallic salts to fluoresce has practical applications because of following reason:
- It is utilized in fluoroscopy, a technique that allows real-time imaging of internal structures by producing visible light when X-rays strike phosphorescent materials.

Q. 39. **Why does computerized tomography (CT) help in the diagnosis of tumors and hemorrhages?**

Answer: Computerized tomography (CT) helps in the diagnosis of tumors and hemorrhages because of following reason:
- It provides detailed cross-sectional images that can reveal the exact location, size, and nature of these abnormalities with high accuracy.

Q. 40. **Why are ultrasonic diagnostic echography procedures considered safe?**

Answer: Ultrasonic diagnostic echography procedures are considered safe because of following reason:
- They use high-frequency sound waves instead of X-rays, which do not pose the same risks of radiation exposure and are non-invasive.

Q. 41. **Why is ultrasound particularly valuable in obstetric and gynecological problems?**
Answer: Ultrasound is particularly valuable in obstetric and gynecological problems because of following reason:
- It allows for the safe and non-invasive monitoring of fetal development.
- The assessment of reproductive organs, provides crucial information without the risks associated with radiation.

Q. 42. **Why might a radiopaque medium be injected during a CT scan?**
Answer: A radiopaque medium might be injected during a CT scan because of following reason:
- It enhances the contrast between vascular and avascular areas, improving the differentiation and visualization of
    - Blood vessels,
    - Tissues, and
    - Abnormalities.

Q. 43. **Why is the AP view preferred for visualizing the thoracic spine?**
Answer: The AP view is preferred for visualizing the thoracic spine because of following reason:
- It aligns the spine closer to the X-ray plate, reducing magnification and distortion.
- It provides a clearer image of the vertebrae and intervertebral discs.

Q. 44. **Why do special views, such as oblique views, exist in radiography? Ai**
Answer: Special views, such as oblique views, exist in radiography because of following reason:
- Certain structures are not well demonstrated in standard views,
- Oblique views helps to provide a more comprehensive assessment of complex anatomical areas.

Q. 45. **Why are dense foreign bodies, like metallic fillings, clearly visible on radiographs?**
Answer: Dense foreign bodies, like metallic fillings, are clearly visible on radiographs because of following reason:
- They are highly radiopaque, meaning they absorb X-rays to a significant degree.
- They create a stark contrast with the surrounding tissues.

11. Vertebral column

General vertebral column

Q. 1. **Why is detailed knowledge of the vertebral column essential to all medical professionals?**
Answer: Detailed knowledge of the vertebral column is essential to all medical professionals because of following reason:
- It affords protection to the spinal cord, supports the trunk, and transmits body weight to the pelvis and lower limbs.

Q. 2. **Why is there an alarming increase in injuries of the vertebral column due to road-traffic accidents? Ai**
Answer: There is an alarming increase in injuries of the vertebral column due to road-traffic accidents because of following reason:
- The impact and trauma sustained during accidents, which affect the structural integrity of the spine.

Q. 3. **Why the vertebral column is considered the axis of the trunk?**
Answer: The vertebral column is considered the axis of the trunk because of following reason:
- It supports the body and provides a central structure to which
  - The trunk and
  - Other body parts are attached.

Q. 4. **Why do the functions of the vertebral column include providing attachment to muscles and ribs?**
Answer: The functions of the vertebral column include providing attachment to muscles and ribs because of following reason:
- This allows for movement and support of the upper body.

Q. 5. **Why is the vertebral foramen important for the passage of spinal nerves?**
Answer: The vertebral foramen is important for the passage of spinal nerves because of following reason:
- It provides a protective canal through which the spinal cord travels and the spinal nerves exit.
- It also plays a role in conditions like disc prolapse.

Q. 6. **Why are the deep muscles of the back important in maintaining the normal curvatures of the vertebral column in the standing position?**

Answer: The deep muscles of the back are important in maintaining the normal curvatures of the vertebral column in the standing position because
- They support the line of gravity passing anterior to the sacrum.

Q. 7. **Why do the erector spinae muscles maintain normal spinal curvature?**

Answer: The erector spinae muscles maintain normal spinal curvature because of following reason:
- By spanning across many vertebrae and adjusting the position of one vertebra to another.

Q. 8. **Why are movements of the vertebral column self-explanatory?**

Answer: Movements of the vertebral column, including flexion, extension, lateral flexion, and rotation, are self-explanatory because of following reason:
- They describe the different ways the spine can move in various directions.

Cervical vertebrae

Q. 9. **Why do cervical, thoracic, and lumbar vertebrae differ from sacral and coccygeal vertebrae in terms of mobility?**

Answer: Cervical, thoracic, and lumbar vertebrae differ from sacral and coccygeal vertebrae in terms of mobility because of following reason:
- Their vertebrae are separate and movable.
- It allows greater flexibility and range of motion.

Q. 10. **Why do the bodies of the vertebrae in the cervical region have saddle-shaped superior surfaces? Ai**

Answer: The bodies of the vertebrae in the cervical region have saddle-shaped superior surfaces because of following reason:
- Their lateral circumference has flange-like lips called uncinate or neurocentral processes, which are their distinguishing feature.

Q. 11. **Why is the odontoid process of the axis vertebra important for the movement of the head?**

Answer: The odontoid process of the axis vertebra is important for the movement of the head because of following reason:
- It acts as a pivot around which the atlas (and thus the head) rotates, allowing for the "yes" (side-to-side) movement of the head.

Q. 12.   **Why does the cervical curvature with convexity facing forwards develop around the age of 3 months?**
Answer: The cervical curvature with convexity facing forwards develops around the age of 3 months because of following reason:
- The infant learns to hold their head erect and directs their visual axes forward.

Thoracic vertebrae

Q. 13.   **Why do the thoracic vertebrae have articular facets on their bodies?**
Answer: The thoracic vertebrae have articular facets on their bodies because of following reason:
- These facets articulate with the ribs, allowing for the attachment and movement of the rib cage.

Q. 14.   **Why do the thoracic vertebrae have vertically oriented zygapophyseal joints?**
Answer: The thoracic vertebrae have vertically oriented zygapophyseal joints because of following reason:
- This orientation limits flexion and extension.
- It facilitates rotational movements of the trunk, which is necessary for activities like twisting and bending.

Q. 15.   **Why are the thoracic and sacral curvatures termed as primary curvatures?**
Answer: The thoracic and sacral curvatures are termed as primary curvatures because of following reason:
- Their curvature direction is the same as the fetal vertebral column, with the concavity facing ventrally.

Q. 16.   **Why are the thoracic and sacral regions termed as primary curvatures?**
Answer: The thoracic and sacral regions are termed as primary curvatures because of following reason:
- Their ventral concavities persist as in prenatal life.

Q. 17.   **Why do the zygapophyseal joints in the thoracic region allow maximum rotation?**
Answer: The zygapophyseal joints in the thoracic region allow maximum rotation because of following reason:
- To compensate for the limitation imposed by the rib cage, which hampers other movements.

Lumbar vertebrae

Q. 18. **Why does the annulus fibrosus consist of many concentric layers of collagenous fibers?**

Answer: The annulus fibrosus consists of many concentric layers of collagenous fibers because of following reason:
- They limit the rotation between vertebrae, thereby providing
  - Stability and
  - Structure to the intervertebral disc.

Q. 19. **Why is the nucleus pulposus of intervertebral discs more posteriorly located in the lumbar region?**

Answer: The nucleus pulposus of intervertebral discs is more posteriorly located in the lumbar region because of following reason:
- It accommodates the greater load-bearing requirements and flexibility needed in the lower back.

Q. 20. **Why is the disc between L4/L5 and L5/S1 more susceptible to disc prolapse in the lumbar region?**

Answer: The disc between L4/L5 and L5/S1 is more susceptible to disc prolapse because of following reason:
- These levels endure significant mechanical stress and movement, increasing the risk of disc herniation.

Q. 21. **Why is disc prolapse more commonly seen in the lumbar region compared to the cervical region?**

Answer: Disc prolapse is more commonly seen in the lumbar region because of following reason:
- The lumbar vertebrae and discs bear more weight and are subject to greater mechanical stresses, increasing the likelihood of disc degeneration and herniation.

Q. 22. **Why does the lumbar curvature with convexity facing forwards develop around the age of 18 months?**

Answer: The lumbar curvature with convexity facing forwards develops around the age of 18 months because of following reason:
- The child acquires the ability to stand and walk erect.

Q. 23. **Why does little rotation occur in the lumbar region?**
Answer: Little rotation occurs in the lumbar region because of following reason:
- Due to the configuration of the zygapophyseal joints, which are oriented to limit rotational movements but allow for flexion, extension, and lateral flexion.

Q. 24. **Why are flexion, extension, and lateral flexion the principal movements of the lumbar spine?**
Answer: Flexion, extension, and lateral flexion are the principal movements of the lumbar spine because of following reason:
- These movements' best suit the anatomical structure and function of the lumbar vertebrae.

Intervertebral discs

Q. 25. **Why does the annulus fibrosus consist of many concentric layers of collagenous fibers?**
Answer: The annulus fibrosus consists of many concentric layers of collagenous fibers because of following reason:
- They limit the rotation between vertebrae, thereby providing
  - Stability and
  - Structure to the intervertebral disc.

Q. 26. **Why is the nucleus pulposus of intervertebral discs more posteriorly located in the lumbar region?**
Answer: The nucleus pulposus of intervertebral discs is more posteriorly located in the lumbar region because of following reason:
- It accommodates the greater load-bearing requirements and flexibility needed in the lower back.

Q. 27. **Why is the disc between L4/L5 and L5/S1 more susceptible to disc prolapse in the lumbar region?**
Answer: The disc between L4/L5 and L5/S1 is more susceptible to disc prolapse because of following reason:
- These levels endure significant mechanical stress and movement, increasing the risk of disc herniation.

Q. 28. **Why is disc prolapse more commonly seen in the lumbar region compared to the cervical region?**

Answer: Disc prolapse is more commonly seen in the lumbar region because of following reason:
- The lumbar vertebrae and discs bear more weight and are subject to greater mechanical stresses, increasing the likelihood of disc degeneration and herniation.

Q. 29. **Why does the lumbar curvature with convexity facing forwards develop around the age of 18 months?**

Answer: The lumbar curvature with convexity facing forwards develops around the age of 18 months because of following reason:
- The child acquires the ability to stand and walk erect.

Q. 30. **Why does little rotation occur in the lumbar region?**

Answer: Little rotation occurs in the lumbar region because of following reason:
- Due to the configuration of the zygapophyseal joints, which are oriented to limit rotational movements but allow for flexion, extension, and lateral flexion.

Q. 31. **Why are flexion, extension, and lateral flexion the principal movements of the lumbar spine?**

Answer: Flexion, extension, and lateral flexion are the principal movements of the lumbar spine because of following reason:
- These movements' best suit the anatomical structure and function of the lumbar vertebrae.

Curvatures of the vertebral column

Q. 32. **Why do the secondary curvatures of the cervical and lumbar regions compensate for the primary curvatures?**

Answer: The secondary curvatures of the cervical and lumbar regions compensate for the primary curvatures because of following reason:
- Their concave direction faces posteriorly, counteracting the primary curvatures.

Q. 33. **Why do kyphosis and lordosis represent abnormal curvatures of the vertebral column?**

Answer: Kyphosis and lordosis represent abnormal curvatures of the vertebral column because of following reason:
- They involve exaggerated convexities either
  - Posteriorly (kyphosis) or
  - Anteriorly (lordosis).

Q. 34. **Why scoliosis is considered an abnormal lateral curvature of the vertebral column?**

Answer: Scoliosis is considered an abnormal lateral curvature of the vertebral column because of following reason:
- It deviates from the normal vertical alignment, either to the right or left.

Miscellaneous questions

Q. 35. **Why are the annulus fibrosus layers of the intervertebral disc arranged in a concentric manner?**

Answer: The annulus fibrosus layers of the intervertebral disc are arranged in a concentric manner because of following reason:
- To limit rotation between the vertebrae.

12. Tendons and ligaments

Tendons

Q. 1. Why are tendons composed of dense fibrous connective tissue containing a high proportion of type I collagen?

Answer: Tendons are composed of dense fibrous connective tissue with a high proportion of type I collagen because of following reason:
- This composition provides them with
    - Strength,
    - Flexibility, and
    - Resilience to withstand the tensile forces exerted by skeletal muscles during movement.

Q. 2. Why can tendons be stretched by 6-15% of their length without damage?

Answer: Tendons can be stretched by 6-15% of their length without damage because of following reason:
- Due to the reorientation of collagen fibers, the straightening of the crimped structure of these fibers, and sliding between adjacent collagen fibrils and fibers.
- This combination allows tendons to accommodate movement without sustaining structural damage.

Q. 3. Why do tendons act as the body's natural shock absorbers during locomotion?

Answer: Tendons act as the body's natural shock absorbers during locomotion because of following reason:
- By storing and releasing strain energy in a rhythmic manner as they stretch and recoil during movement.
- This helps in smoothening the movement and reduces the impact forces transmitted to the skeletal system, minimizing the risk of injury.

Q. 4. Why do tendons rarely receive a blood supply across their osseotendinous junctions?

Answer: Tendons rarely receive a blood supply across their osseotendinous junctions because of following reason:
- Blood vessels rarely pass between bone and tendon at these attachments, and the junctional surfaces are usually devoid of foramina.
- Exceptions include the calcaneal (Achilles) tendon, which does receive a blood supply across its osseotendinous junction.

Q. 5. Why do tendons not recover their original strength completely after repair?

Answer: Tendons do not recover their original strength completely after repair because of following reason:
- Complete turnover (replacement) of the tissue, as seen in bone, does not occur in adult tendons.
- Therefore, healed tendons do not regain the same structural integrity and strength as their original state, even after repair processes involving fibroblast proliferation and collagen fiber deposition.

Q. 6. Why do tendons consist of longitudinally arranged collagen fibers?

Answer: Tendons consist of longitudinally arranged collagen fibers because of following reason:
- This structure provides them with strength and flexibility, enabling them to transmit the force generated by muscles to bones.

Q. 7. Why are tendons supplied with blood from multiple sources?

Answer: Tendons are supplied with blood from multiple sources because of following reason:
- They require a rich blood supply to maintain their integrity and repair any damage incurred during movement or stress.

Q. 8. Why do tendons passing around loops or pulleys have synovial sheaths?

Answer: Tendons passing around loops or pulleys have synovial sheaths because of following reason:
- To help lubricate the tendon, reducing friction.
- They allow smooth movement, especially in areas of high stress or repetitive motion.

Q. 9. Why do synovial sheaths have visceral and parietal layers?

Answer: Synovial sheaths have visceral and parietal layers because of following reason:
- To facilitate smooth movement of the tendon within the sheath.
- The visceral layer is firmly attached to the tendon, while the parietal layer is attached to surrounding structures, allowing them to glide on each other.

Q. 10. Why do some tendons have mesotendon or vinculum?

Answer: Some tendons have mesotendon or vinculum because of following reason: Blood vessels perforate the synovial sheath, forming a fold that supports blood supply to the tendon.
- This arrangement helps reinforce the longitudinal anastomosis.
- It provides additional nourishment to the tendon.

Q. 11. **Why are sesamoid fibrocartilages common in tendons or joint capsules?**

Answer: Sesamoid fibrocartilages are common in tendons or joint capsules because of following reason:
- They help reduce friction.
- They provide a smooth surface for tendons to glide over bony prominences during movement.

Q. 12. **Why is the ossification of some sesamoid fibrocartilages considered a mystery?**

Answer: The ossification of some sesamoid fibrocartilages is considered a mystery because of following reason:
- The reasons behind why certain sesamoid bones develop and ossify while others remain fibrocartilaginous are not fully understood.

Q. 13. **Why are the tendons arranged in a specific order on the dorsal aspect of the wrist?**

Answer: The tendons on the dorsal aspect of the wrist because of following reason:
- Arranged in a specific order from lateral to medial.
- It provide a clear pathway for
    - Muscle movements and
    - To prevent friction and overlap, ensuring smooth extension and flexion of the wrist and fingers.

Q. 14. **Why is Gruber's Bursa significant in the musculoskeletal system?**

Answer: Gruber's Bursa is significant in the musculoskeletal system because of following reason:
- It reduces friction between
    - The tendons of the extensor digitorum longus and
    - The head of the talus, playing a role in smooth foot movements.

Q. 15. **Why is Parona's space relevant in forearm anatomy?**

Answer: Parona's space is relevant in forearm anatomy because of following reason:
- It is a fascial interval deep to the flexor tendons, indicating its significance in forearm infections and compartment syndrome.

Q. 16. **Why is the pulse of the posterior tibial artery felt between the tendons of flexor digitorum longus and flexor hallucis longus?**

Answer: The posterior tibial artery is palpable at this location because of following reason:
- It passes deep to the flexor retinaculum and between these tendons as it descends towards the foot.

Q. 17. **Why do sesamoid bones develop in muscle tendons and lack periosteum and Haversian systems?**

Answer: Sesamoid bones develop in muscle tendons and lack periosteum and Haversian systems because of following reason:
- To provide a mechanical advantage by reducing friction and increasing the leverage of the muscle.
- They lack periosteum and Haversian systems because their primary function is to enhance tendon movement and efficiency rather than support weight or facilitate nutrient supply.

Q. 18. **Why is the anatomical zone of injury in the hand called no man's land?**

Answer: The anatomical zone of injury in the hand is called no man's land because of following reason:
- Zone 2 of the finger, which has a snug sheath around two tendons, is critical for
    - Prognosis and
    - Management of flexor tendon injuries, making it a challenging area for surgical repair.

Q. 19. **Why do ruptured tendons take a long time to heal?**

Answer: Ruptured tendons take a long time to heal because of following reason:
- They have few blood vessels entering their substance.
- It results, delay in reaching the nutrients, chemicals, and cells essential for tissue repair.
- There is, prolongation of the healing process.

Ligaments

Q. 20. **Why are ligaments essential in preventing abnormal movements of joints?**

Answer: Ligaments are essential in preventing abnormal movements of joints because of following reason:
- Their tough and unyielding nature restricts movements beyond the normal range, protecting the joint from injuries.

Q. 21. Why are intrinsic ligaments significant in joint anatomy?
Answer: Intrinsic ligaments are significant in joint anatomy because of following reason:
- They surround the joint, providing additional support and stability.
- They can be either extracapsular or intracapsular depending on their specific location.

Q. 22. Why do ligaments have a rich nerve supply?
Answer: Ligaments have a rich nerve supply because of following reason:
- Their sensory function is critical for detecting joint position and movement.
- It helps in maintaining joint stability through reflex actions.

Q. 23. Why do ligaments vary in their composition of collagen and elastin fibers?
Answer: Ligaments vary in their composition of collagen and elastin fibers because of following reason:
- Different joints require different levels of flexibility and strength.
- The collagen provides toughness.
- The elastin providing stretchability where needed.

Q. 24. Why is the sensory function of ligaments important for their role in joint stability?
Answer: The sensory function of ligaments is important for their role in joint stability because of following reason:
- It enables them to act as reflex organs.
- It enhances their ability to respond to changes in joint position and movement efficiently.

Q. 25. Why do torn ligaments destabilize joints and increase the risk of dislocation?
Answer: Torn ligaments destabilize joints and increase the risk of dislocation because of following reason:
- They weaken the structural integrity of the joint, compromising its stability. Hence, joints with torn ligaments are more prone to dislocation.

www.ingramcontent.com/pod-product-compliance
Lightning Source LLC
Chambersburg PA
CBHW062101220526
45471CB00010B/3563